"Fanny Brewster throws open the doors of the slave quarters, casts light on the face of unbearable grief, rage and intergenerational trauma. She insists we remember what the culture, and indeed, Depth Psychology, has preferred to forget—the appalling cruelty and systemic evil of American slavery during the 400 years of the African Holocaust, how its social and psychological legacy shapes our world to this day.

The Ancestors speak to Brewster, especially 'mothering slaves'—women forced to be 'breeders,' whose labor in childbirth and in the cotton fields brought them no joy, no increase, no profit. Their bodies were not their own; they were used and abused. Their children were not their own; they were ripped from their breasts. Their families were not their own; they were torn apart. They tell Motherline stories from hell.

Archetypal Grief is strong medicine for the soul. If your heart is open to sorrow, to horror, if your mind is open to seeing through cultural complexes and denial, if your ears are open to 'the voice of the Other,' if you long for healing, if you want to 'be woke,' this book is for you."

—**Naomi Ruth Lowinsky**, author of *The Motherline: Every Woman's Journey to Find Her Female Roots* and *The Rabbi, the Goddesss and Jung: Getting the Word from Within*

"Dr. Brewster advances the argument that we, 'both whites and blacks,' are haunted by the '*not* telling' of the historical slave stories and their continuing archetypal manifestations. White America, in Dr. Martin Luther King, Jr.'s words, is 'poisoned to its soul' by racism, and we are equally haunted by *not* listening to our black sisters and brothers, past and present. Such listening would be one way to help purge our souls of racism's poison through empathetic witnessing, a form of *archetypal apology*, if you will. To do so, we need to counter white fragility by having the strength to turn the pages of books like *Archetypal Grief,* and not look away from the anguish and anger therein, nor deny our ancestors' roles in their genesis and the *archetypal guilt* we carry in our DNA as well."

—**Jennifer Leigh Selig, PhD**, author of *Integration: The Psychology and Mythology of Martin Luther King, Jr. and His (Unfinished) Therapy With the Soul of America*

"You birth a child and they die because you are malnourished. You birth a child knowing they are the product of a rape. You birth a child and at adolescence they are maimed, tortured or flogged to death. You birth a child and they are torn from your arms and sold you know not where.

This is the archetypal legacy of the African Holocaust explored by Jungian analyst Dr. Fanny Brewster who challenges us to become conscious of the grief, sorrow, rage as well as the strength and resilience experienced and embedded in the emotional DNA of those *'mothering slaves'* and handed down to their descendants. The trauma of this legacy affects all and is embedded in all our psyches.

Bring your heart and your soul, your emotions as well as your intellect as you read this searing, scholarly work."

—**Christine M. Chao, PhD**, clinical psychologist,
diplomate Jungian analyst, USA

"Fanny Brewster provides a necessary exploration of the impact on African-Americans of a devastating evil of slavery, the tearing of children away from their mothers. She writes with passion and power, using the lens of Jungian archetypes in conjunction with her profound understanding of African-American culture, to decipher the complexities of slavery's aftermath. Considering past, future, and spiritual integrity, she leads us to an understanding of feelings that still reverberate, archetypal grief as a steady-state, pervasive element over a lifetime, within a culture of resilience and survival."

—**Merle Molofsky, NCPsyA, LP**, psychoanalyst, faculty member and Advisory Board, Harlem Family Institute, USA; faculty member, NPAP

ARCHETYPAL GRIEF

Archetypal Grief: Slavery's Legacy of Intergenerational Child Loss is a powerful exploration of the intergenerational psychological effects of child loss as experienced by women held in slavery in the Americas and of its ongoing effects in contemporary society. It presents the concept of archetypal grief in African American women: cultural trauma so deeply wounding that it spans generations.

Calling on Jungian psychology as well as neuroscience and attachment theory, Fanny Brewster explores the psychological lives of enslaved women using their own narratives and those of their descendants, and discusses the stories of mothering slaves with reference to their physical and emotional experiences. The broader context of slavery and the conditions leading to the development of archetypal grief are examined, with topics including the visibility/invisibility of the African female body, the archetype of the mother, stereotypes about black women, and the significance of rites of passage. The discussion is placed in the context of contemporary America and the economic, educational, spiritual and political legacy of slavery.

Archetypal Grief will be an important work for academics and students of Jungian and post-Jungian studies, archetypal and depth psychology, archetypal studies, feminine psychology, women's studies, the history of slavery, African American history, African diaspora studies and sociology. It will also be of interest to analytical psychologists and Jungian psychotherapists in practice and in training.

Fanny Brewster, PhD, is a Jungian analyst and Professor at Pacifica Graduate Institute, USA. She is the author of *African Americans and Jungian Psychology: Leaving the Shadows* (Routledge, 2017).

ARCHETYPAL GRIEF

Slavery's Legacy of Intergenerational Child Loss

Fanny Brewster

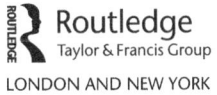

LONDON AND NEW YORK

First published 2019
by Routledge
2 Park Square, Milton Park, Abingdon, Oxon OX14 4RN

and by Routledge
711 Third Avenue, New York, NY 10017

Routledge is an imprint of the Taylor & Francis Group, an informa business

© 2019 Fanny Brewster

The right of Fanny Brewster to be identified as the author of this work has been asserted by her in accordance with sections 77 and 78 of the Copyright, Designs and Patents Act 1988.

All rights reserved. No part of this book may be reprinted or reproduced or utilised in any form or by any electronic, mechanical, or other means, now known or hereafter invented, including photocopying and recording, or in any information storage or retrieval system, without permission in writing from the publishers.

Trademark notice: Product or corporate names may be trademarks or registered trademarks, and are used only for identification and explanation without intent to infringe.

British Library Cataloguing in Publication Data
A catalogue record for this book is available from the British Library

Library of Congress Cataloging in Publication Data
Names: Brewster, Fanny, author.
Title: Archetypal grief : slavery's legacy of intergenerational child loss / Fanny Brewster.
Description: 1 Edition. | New York : Routledge, 2019.
Identifiers: LCCN 2018019022| ISBN 9780415789059 (hardback) | ISBN 9780415789066 (pbk.) | ISBN 9781315222998 (ebook)
Subjects: LCSH: Loss (Psychology)--United States--History. | Mother and child--United States--History. | Separation anxiety--United States--History. | Slavery--United States--History. | Jungian psychology--United States--History.
Classification: LCC BF575.D35 B74 2019 | DDC 155.9/3--dc23
LC record available at https://lccn.loc.gov/2018019022

ISBN: 978-0-415-78905-9 (hbk)
ISBN: 978-0-415-78906-6 (pbk)
ISBN: 978-1-315-22299-8 (ebk)

Typeset in Bembo
by Taylor & Francis Books

Dedicated to my Mother and Foremothers

CONTENTS

Acknowledgements   *x*
Foreword   *xii*
Introduction   *xx*

1   Archetypes of the collective unconscious   1

2   The mother archetype   8

3   Rites of passage: Life and death   18

4   Slavery as archetype and the prayer of freedom   28

5   Mothering slave and the intergenerational orphan   41

6   African Americans and Elisabeth Kübler-Ross: Stages of grief   54

7   Grief as anger   68

8   Archetypal grief   82

9   Mother, daughter, son   96

10   The female Africanist body   110

11   Mirror as symbol   120

12   Influencing the archetype   127

Summary   134

References   *139*
Index   *143*

ACKNOWLEDGEMENTS

I wish to thank friends, colleagues and family who gave me support before and during the writing of *Archetypal Grief: Slavery's Legacy of Intergenerational Child Loss*.

Dr. Julie Bondanza provided guidance through much of my clinical experience in preparation to become a Jungian analyst and clinical psychologist. I am grateful to have received her humorous and clearly focused direction on how to just *be*, in and with that process.

Women writer-friends have provided me with support as I complained, cried and engaged with the material of this book. Robin Grice, Lauren Sallinger, Marisa Novello and Magin LaSov Gregg. We have been initiated together as writers and I am very grateful to have them for comfort and support as writer-friends.

I met Valerie Hummingbird several years ago at the Omega Institute in Rhinebeck, New York, at a writer's retreat and she gave me a fertility amulet from Niger. I thank her for her gracious kindness to me that day.

My community of Philadelphia Jungian analysts (PAJA) has been a strong source of support for me in my analytical life and I am most appreciative of this support.

Helen Palmer was able to share a vision for my life as a writer when I could barely perceive of one. I thank her for what she saw in me and for all that she has given to me.

Dianne Travis-Teague, Alumni Director at Pacifica Graduate Institute, has shown great support for me as a writer, teacher, and friend within the Pacifica community. I am most grateful for her presence in my life.

I thank Andrew Samuels for his political activism and its influential support of me as a writer.

The San Francisco Jungian analyst community invited me to their Institute where I first presented a paper on "Archetypal Grief in African American Women." I am exceedingly thankful to them for their invitation and warm reception that encouraged me to develop that paper into *Archetypal Grief: Slavery's Legacy of Intergenerational Child Loss*.

Heather Formaini had the courage to present my speech at the IAAP Jungian activism gathering in Prague when I could not be there in person. I appreciate her willingness to stand with me in solidarity.

I first met Inez Martinez a few years ago at the C. G. Jung Foundation in New York where I was presenting a workshop on Odysseus. I am very pleased that she has agreed to write the Foreword for this book and I thank her.

Susannah Frearson, Editor at Routledge, has provided sincere and excellent editorial direction for which I am grateful.

FOREWORD

Fanny Brewster's *Archetypal Grief: Slavery's Legacy of Intergenerational Child Loss*, an imaginative rendering of the suffering of African slaves in America and of their African American descendants, appears at a pivotal moment in the unfolding of American history. Brewster's book brings light to buried horror at the very historical moment that Americans are being forced to struggle with our past. Claims of advocates of white supremacy have erupted into mainstream public consciousness through the elevation to the presidency of Donald Trump, demagogical promoter of exclusionary policies and apologist for racist protestors. Trump's ascent to power, because it implicitly bestows legitimacy on the idea that white people are superior and should dominate others, shoves into public consciousness the long-repressed roots of this claim: the historical practice of white colonists and Americans of enacting a presumed right to buy, own, chain, work, sell, rape, whip, maim, and, if they wished, kill black people first stolen from Africa, then bred like livestock for profit.

Archetypal Grief shares Brewster's active imagination of the psychological legacy of what Samuel Kimbles has called "social suffering" (2014, p. 2) being lived by descendants of American slavery. Her empathic projections of herself into how life has felt to generations of African Americans is informed by transdisciplinary research not only into psychological structures, myth, and neuroscience, but also into history seen through slave narratives and anthropological studies of African cultures.

Her book is well read in tandem with Kimbles' *Phantom Narratives:* The Unseen Contributions of Culture to Psyche. Kimbles' contribution of the idea of *phantom narratives*, that is, intergenerational unconscious processes manifesting in 'unresolved or unworked-through grief and violence that occurred in a prior historical cultural context and continues into the present' (2014, p. 21), provides a theoretical framework for reading Brewster's resurrecting of her ancestors' suffering. Brewster, as the title of her book indicates, chooses to frame her work through the concept of the archetype. I believe she chooses *archetypal* to summon a sense of the transcendence of time and the depth of the grief. Placing the depth at the level of the archetype raises the question of whether the grief can be relieved, a question Brewster, herself, wonders about in thinking of the violence of racism. Her entire work, however, exists as an effort to begin to heal that grief. My sense is that the term *phantom* better suits her intentions, a point to which I will return when suggesting the kind of future work *Archetypal Grief* opens up.

Brewster's meditations on the suffering borne by Africans and its continuation in the generations of their descendants is a first step toward fulfillment of the requirements for healing. Trauma specialist Betty P. Teng describes the traumatized victim as speechless and needing language expressing what has happened as a first step, then having that expression witnessed and affirmed as real (2017, pp. 225–226, 229). She describes how in therapy, safe space for that mourning is offered. There is no office or therapist for the expressing and witnessing of group trauma such as enslavement. Brewster emphasizes the consequent invisibility of what she terms the holocaust of Africans during slavery. Her effort to give voice to the suffering of African American slaves still haunting their descendants is thus an effort to find a way to help to heal a group trauma. I experience her articulation of the suppressed psychological pain of the enslaved as also providing an opportunity for reconceiving the American dream. The current resurfacing of the claims of white supremacy into public discourse threatens the humane aspect of that dream. In its ideal form, the dream of "America" is the vision of developing a society of free persons with equal rights seeking to organize themselves in a socially just and personally enabling way. This dream has been historically impeded and morally betrayed by its failure to accord full human status to all human groups and thus to recognize human interconnectedness and interdependence. Brewster's detailing of the psychological griefs of enslaved Africans and their descendants offers the rest of Americans the opportunity to experience social suffering as we recognize this atrocity in our history and begin to experience responsibility for the benefits of the lives we live as its aftermath—more relatedly, as we begin to be able to empathize with the grief felt by our fellow and sister human beings.

Since Brewster is attempting to illuminate an emotion, horrendous grief, her writing circles, touching again and again in different contexts, on particular wounds. The one to which she returns most often and from most perspectives is that of the black woman, her experience of mothering, of being a body, of having her cultural understanding of procreation violently denied her. Brewster places the suffering of black mother slaves in the context of the archetype of the Mother of Sorrows. She grounds that pain in reflections on the slave mother's helplessness with regard to being bred, raped and deprived of her children forever when they were sold off. Throughout her reflections, Brewster attempts to understand the kind of suffering emanating from the loss of homeland and culture, thus refuting the slavers' rationalization that Africans had no philosophy or vision of life's meaning. Thinking of the suffering of slave mothers, for example, she cites an

African belief in reincarnation that valued procreation as part of the cycle of life and death (see Chapter 3 in this volume):

> The accompanying mourning and celebration for each new death and each birth were acknowledged as reflections of the continuous lives of ancestors entering and leaving the same space. The Beng people have a word—*wrugbe*—which translates as spirit village. This is the place where souls return after death and also the place from where the souls of children leave to enter earth-bound lives.

Imagining herself into the experience of her slave ancestors, Brewster offers to her readers an instance of what kind of suffering the loss of their culture inflicted: slave mothers having their reproductive lives turned into being bred like domesticated animals, depriving them not only of their human right to mother their children, but of their human right to fulfill a religious understanding of their role in the drama of life and death. Her book is lit with such moments of cultural understanding and opportunity for readers who are not descendants of African slaves empathically to share the humanity and grief of American enslaved foremothers.

This book is not a comfortable read for non-descendants of African American slaves. It reveals an ugly shadow of Americans' celebration of the uniqueness of American commitment to freedom. Winning the war of independence from Great Britain in the name of the equal rights of man and proclaiming the American government a republic formed by "freemen" paradoxically further normalized the dehumanizing of slaves through the uniting of whiteness and freedom. David R. Roediger's *The Wages of Whiteness* details the history of white men in America coping with the economic facts that urbanization meant America would not consist primarily of independent farmers as in Jefferson's vision of free Americans. Instead, workers were becoming increasingly dependent on employers willing to provide jobs, a dilemma still undermining the independence of American workers. A mainstay of these workers seeking to maintain their self-respect as they lost autonomy consisted of comparing themselves favorably against slaves. White men might be "hirelings," but would never be dehumanized into chattel. This relative state of freedom was increasingly defended vigorously in terms of color by workers and used as a form of reimbursement or "wages" by employers (Roediger, 1991, p. 137). The arrogation of freedom and power to whiteness and assignment of enslavement and subjugation to blackness form part of the phantom narrative continuing to produce social suffering in America. Brewster calls for a reimagining of freedom, and by implication suggests that understanding the role of *psychological* freedom from complexes and from haunting phantoms is fundamental to any such reimagining.

Understanding this vision requires understanding the controlling power of complexes. In *Phantom Narratives* Kimbles explains the development of the ideas of cultural unconsciousness, cultural complexes, and phantom narratives, and he begins with a history of Jung's concept of the complex. Based on patients' patterns of hesitations during word association tests, Jung deduced that a person's unconscious contains "splinter psyches" ([1934] 1960, para. 203) that exist alongside the ego which normally can choose among possible responses. He called these autonomous "splinter psyches" complexes and thought of them as having the power to take over the ego's role without an individual knowing that it is happening. Once a complex replaces the organizing function of the ego, a person's response is predictable because it no longer has even the relative freedom of normal consciousness.

Someone suffering a victim complex, for example, will experience life's challenges as victimization, a situation explored by James Baldwin in his short story, "Sonny's Blues." This complex is particularly difficult to overcome when external life indeed is in many ways victimizing one. Sonny, a black son of Harlem, caught in living life as a victim of a racist society, seeks to escape suffering through taking drugs. In prison, trapped in a cell with his "own stink" (Baldwin, 1965, p. 116), he learns to take responsibility for himself through recognizing the role of his agency in his suffering. He thus escapes filtering all his experiences through identifying as a victim, gaining increasing psychological freedom from the control of his complex. This development of consciousness enables him to turn his own suffering and that of his ancestors into the transformative music of Blues. Part of the work of therapy consists of assisting analysands to become conscious when in the grips of a complex.

Jung thought of complexes as living units in the unconscious of individuals. Joseph Henderson introduced the idea of a realm of unconscious psyche between the archetypal (universal) and personal (unique) dimensions—the cultural unconscious. In giving this history, Kimbles acknowledges his role in adding dynamics to the idea of the cultural unconscious by conceptualizing cultural complexes. He conceives them as structures that organize common human needs: "Cultural complexes are a dynamic system of relations that serve the basic need for belonging and identity through linking personal experiences and group expectations as these are mediated by ethnicity, race, religion, and gender processes" (2014, p. 5). Adding the dynamism of the complex theoretically supports hope of group susceptibility to transformation. To this multi-level understanding of the unconscious psyche, Kimbles adds the idea of *phantom narratives*, phantoms because like ghosts they are not materially there but are nevertheless present. He writes, "My first hypothesis then is that intergenerational processes are manifested as phantom narratives that provide structure, representation, and continuity for unresolved or unworked-through grief and violence that occurred in a prior historical cultural context and continues into the present" (ibid., p. 21). What Kimbles is calling a phantom narrative is precisely what Brewster through active imagination and research is making visible so that it can be witnessed in order to begin the process of healing. Healing would mean greater psychological freedom both for the descendants of slaves and for those readers empathically participating through their own development of consciousness.

Brewster and Kimbles' work continues the effort of Jung to account for human beings being unconsciously controlled by the past, an effort crystallized in his concept of the archetype. For those unfamiliar with that concept, Jung sought psychological and cultural images of experiences common to all humankind no matter the era, experiences such as being parented, being a child, encountering a gendered Other, and acting in evil ways. He speculated that the potential for certain patterning of those experiences which he called *archetypes* was unconsciously shared by all human beings, resulting in what he explored as mother, father, and child archetypes with regard to parenting; anima and animus archetypes with regard to experiencing gendered Others; and the shadow archetype with regard to humans enacting evil. Archetypes manifesting in human behavior are the presence of the past in human behavior in any era.

The characteristic of an archetype important for understanding Brewster's book is that, like complexes, as an unconscious force an archetype can overwhelm consciousness and take over. Unlike complexes, however, an archetype is not just an unconscious force in an individual or in a cultural group, but in psyche, itself, like a kind of psychic DNA conveyed through the history of all humanity to each human being. A major task of individual consciousness, or the ego, is to develop a relationship with the archetypes unconsciously affecting the individual and not to identify with them. Identifying means becoming possessed by them and losing the possibility of rational discrimination. Jung analyzes German participation in Nazi warlikeness in these terms. Being overwhelmed by an archetype is like living a fate. That is why it matters whether an evil inflicted by a group is a manifestation of shadow which is an archetypal unconscious force, or of a cultural complex. If a behavior pattern is the result of a cultural complex, the goal of cultural transformation through the development of consciousness becomes, at least theoretically, a more realizable undertaking.

As Brewster delves into her ancestral past, she makes use of all three concepts, *archetypal, cultural complex, and phantom* and ties them to the soul of African Americans (see Chapter 7 in this volume):

> African Americans are within a cultural complex that holds not only the positive images and dynamism of their individual lives but also those of the group. This group dynamic also contains the phantoms of the past lives of those who have preceded them. The connections between those who have passed into death and those who remain are connected on an archetypal level that brings into a cultural reality the soul of the group.

She thus draws upon Jungian and post-Jungian theorizing as she continues the work of seeking psychological freedom from the constraints of the past.

Another reason Brewster's book challenges sympathetic reading is that, like many a black woman writer before her, (see, for example, Guy-Sheftall, 1995), she defends the right of the traumatized to experience and assert anger. She criticizes the negative attitude of the dominant culture toward the "angry black woman." She identifies with the causes of the anger of black women, including their contemporaneous worry about the dominant culture's hostility toward black men manifested in the rate of their incarceration vis-à-vis white men and their killing by police. She unequivocally calls for acceptance of the appropriateness of their anger, asserting: "anger is [the black woman's] privilege and right, claimed through generations of grief she has had to carry." In the protective confines of the therapist's office, getting in touch with anger and expressing it is often an essential step in moving from being caught in a complex to having more options about how to respond when encountering experiences touching the complex. In the public arena, however, anger is resisted as threatening and destructive. One of the challenges Brewster's presentation of the grief of African Americans brings to collective consciousness is the task of how to structure, witness, contain, and allow the work of anger to take place in the collective healing process. Truth commissions have been tried in over a dozen nations with varying, mostly minimal, levels of success to heal divided societies. Brewster's use of active imagination to bring the emotions of traumatized ancestors to consciousness in a book available to all who can read can be viewed as an attempt to provide a social structure for the necessary step of expressing and validating group anger. Her book expresses that anger, and the reception of her book will determine whether that approach results in the anger being validated so that healing can proceed.

One possible validation would consist of future work in imitation of her modeling the articulation of a phantom narrative. *Archetypal Grief* paves the way for other spokespersons to reflect on the phantom narratives of their ancestors, descendants of Native Americans, for example. Such articulations would contribute to the collective self-knowledge needed for pursuing the American dream in its ideal form. *Archetypal Grief* inspires research in other ways as well. Brewster often punctuates her reflections with a series of questions that open up areas of inquiry to bring to consciousness complexes fixating our cultural relations and behavior in social suffering. For example, after having repeatedly encountered depression in her analysands, and after having imagined an ongoing state of depression suffered by slaves (one that arguably *requires* manifestation of anger), she asks (see Chapter 6 in this volume):

> What is the consistent and frequent healing that would have supported a letting go of this type of depression? How have we as a cultural group begun to have enough of the conversations regarding group healing [for] this level of cultural trauma [to] heal? What would it take for such a beginning and engagement with healing to commence?

As hinted earlier, another direction for future work emerges from the incompletely differentiated relations of the terms *archetypal, complex,* and *phantom narrative.* Brewster, herself, only occasionally uses the term *phantom* although Kimbles' concept arguably presents the most persuasive image for intergenerational continuity of group traumas. The meaning of the term "archetypal" has been complicated by James Hillman's taking it to describe his vision of psychology. Hillman acknowledges Jung's conception of archetypes as transcendent proto-forms, but appropriates the term to refer to phenomenal images of psyche conceived as an imaginal realm. He believes that through imaginative engagement with the world, soul is created: "the aim of therapy .... is the development of a sense of soul, the middle ground of psychic realities, and the method of therapy is the cultivation of imagination" (1983, p. 4). Although Brewster cites passages from Jung describing archetypes, her relationship to the idea of the archetypal seems rooted in Hillman's vision because, as her title, *Archetypal Grief*, announces, she finds the archetypal in emotions, a move justified in Hillman's claim that the concept "archetypal belongs to all culture" (ibid., p. 1). As indicated earlier, she sees the connections between "those who have passed into death and those who remain" existing on "an archetypal level that brings into a cultural reality the soul of the group." Expansion of the discursive realm of archetypes is problematic because perceived manifestations of archetypes in cultures can be and have been treated as naturalizations of what are in fact cultural expressions. Brewster's suggestion that slavery is an archetype, for example, using Jung's understanding of *archetypal*, discursively leads to an assumption that it always has been and always will be a social form of power that humans use. Efforts such as Brewster's to heal the psychological wounds of the descendants of slavery make sense in a vision of human history in the process of realizing, in the aphorism popularized by Dr. Martin Luther King, an arc bending toward social justice. Her desire to communicate the intergenerational character of the emotion of grief and its susceptibility to transformation seem to me better expressed through the concepts of the cultural complex and the phantom narrative which are open to amelioration through time through consciousness. In any case, Brewster's book helps to bring into focus the need for Jungian and post-Jungian scholars to clarify the relations between and use of the terms *archetypal, cultural complex,* and *phantom narrative.*

Brewster's book also specifically challenges the Jungian community to undertake the work of professionally acknowledging its unconsciousness with regard to many beliefs that affect people of color in America differently than they affect white people. Jung's use of a framework of opposites, for example, supports collective "othering" of the disempowered by dominant groups. She suggests that it's the white lens of European culture that allows theorizing myths concerning gods and goddesses as expressions of the unconscious psyche, but not dreams or visions of ancestors. She asks for analysis of white rage. She acknowledges that she personally received racist responses during her training to become a Jungian analyst. She calls for Jungians to recognize that "color does matter," to apply their willingness to look into the "dark places of psyche," that is, their own unconscious lens of whiteness to discover *how* color matters and to integrate that understanding into their professional activities as teachers and healers. Simultaneously, Brewster insists on the necessity of self-definition of groups rendered invisible by whiteness. She offers her book imagining the intergenerational experience of grief stemming from enslavement as an example of such self-definition emerging from the journey of descendants of African American slavery toward psychological freedom.

The ongoing racism suffered by Americans, brought to a crisis demanding consciousness through the permission given to white supremacists again to make their claims in the public forum through the presidency of Donald Trump, testifies to the insolubility of value conflicts through force. The question of whether whites are inherently entitled to subjugate blacks and other people of color was not settled psychologically by the North's winning the Civil War nor by Lincoln's proclaiming the end of slavery. Alabama's Republican candidate for the United States Senate in 2018, more than 150 years since the end of the American Civil War over slavery, publicly proclaimed that America was last great during the days of slavery. Such struggles over issues of power cannot be resolved by power. They require imaginative responses, the development of what Andrew Samuels has called "moral imagination" (1986, p. 73) that can transform unconscious attitudes. Art is one imaginative response, and it has offered visions of how to transform the complex issuing from racism in works such as James Baldwin's short story, "Sonny's Blues," Toni Morrison's novel, *Beloved*, and Maya Angelou's poem, "And Still I Rise." Fanny Brewster's conveying of the grief of the descendants of African American slaves offers the way of historical, cultural imagining to help to relieve their social suffering. It simultaneously offers other Americans an opportunity not only to bear witness to that suffering, but to experience grief over and repudiation of slavery. Brewster seeks collective expression of remorse. She also affirms the power of descendants of American slaves to forgive. Writing *Archetypal Grief* puts her in the line of ancestors of all colors who have sought to convey a vision of justice and freedom, in this case psychological freedom, through understanding suffering.

Inez Martinez

INTRODUCTION

> Nobody ever helps me into carriages, or over mud-puddles, or gives me any best place! And ain't I a woman? Look at me! Look at my arm! I have ploughed and planted, and gathered into barns, and no man could head me! And ain't I a woman? I could work as much and eat as much as a man—when I could get it—and bear the lash as well! And ain't I a woman? I have borne thirteen children, and seen most all sold off to slavery, and when I cried out with my mother's grief, none but Jesus heard me! And ain't I a woman?
>
> Sojourner Truth, May 29, 1851 (White, 1998, p. 14)

Women of color have given birth to children for centuries, raising and loving them through the most arduous and humanly painful circumstances. Birthing and raising children through slavery, being a mothering slave, is one of these circumstances in which millions of African diaspora women both survived and died during the time of the African Holocaust—slavery in the Southern plantation system. Today, we might think less frequently about the facts of slavery and its impact on African American women. We may have a tendency towards acknowledging that American slavery existed, but also think, why not just move on—let the past be forgotten. This is unfortunately one of the main features of our American social narrative regarding slavery and its effects. Memories of those of Africanist ancestry have been lost, stolen and distorted, oftentimes beyond recognition. The important necessary work is in the questioning and recovery of the memory of those who lived through and after slavery.

It is important because our past continues to live with and sometimes haunt us in the present time. I believe this is especially true in terms of mother-child relationships. *Archetypal Grief: Slavery's Legacy of Intergenerational Child Loss* is about the conscious and unconscious grief and sorrow borne for centuries by women of color due to slavery. This is specifically related to American slavery, yet generally connects all women of color where European slavery influenced and destroyed maternal-child relationships and lives, during colonial and post-colonial times. It is specifically related to the psychological lives of women of color whether they birth children into the world or choose not to have biological children. Another important reason that I say our past continues to haunt us is because we carry from one generation to the next the archetypal DNA of unconscious processes that influence us in ways we continue to discover in the 21st century.

Neuroscience has opened up the discussions regarding the long-held view of the archetypes and the collective unconscious as first proposed by not only Jung, but others before him. The status of our brain functioning includes the necessary importance of memory recall. This ability to carry memory on both conscious and unconscious levels helps us to connect and bond with each other first in early childhood, and later in relationships beyond the childhood home. It is the memories of those early relationships that help to form us and create "models" for future patterns of behavior. How do these models influence what we believe about ourselves, and those in our American collective?

Perhaps we are seeing more into what motivates us, controls us and predicts who we are as human beings, as concepts such as mirroring neurons and the theories of the effects of Attachment Disorder become more commonplace in our psychological and broad social settings. Attachment Theory gives a perspective on how we bond and become relational with others in those early infant and childhood years. How did the children of mothering slaves feel and grow in terms of bonding and attachment? In *Archetypal Grief: Slavery's Legacy of Intergenerational Child Loss*, the Emotional Body is considered as well as the female Africanist body since so much of our conversation regarding grief is centered on this feminine body. It is interesting to note that in my review of material for writing this book, there has been almost a total absence of historical authors making mention of the emotional impact of slavery on mothering slaves.

I would say our past continues with us as Sam Kimbles in *Phantom Narratives: The Unseen Contributions of Culture to Psyche*, has described because we live with the results of American slavery and its intergenerational racial effect on the lives of African Americans in this contemporary life. We witness this effect daily. Almost each day, somewhere in America, we see played out over and again the results of slavery and the price African Americans have paid through the suffering lives of each new generation.

This payment is economic, educational, spiritual as well as physical. Sometimes the payment takes the form of the loss of a child's life. A mother's unconscious hidden fear is realized. Other times the price is the nagging, worrying anxiety of struggling to protect your African American child within a society where his or her preciousness is severely restricted by skin color.

The African American mother can think: will my teenage son or daughter remember that when faced with a possible deadly situation away from the safety of our home, their ethnicity could mean life or death? Will they make the choice that brings them safely home to me? There is no manner in which slavery has not been a painfully horrible intrusion into the lives of African Americans as individuals, families and communities.

The grief of knowing that one is a breeder of children for the economic success of a plantation system is an unimaginable horror. Yet this is the way millions of African American women lived for centuries—knowing that their children were never going to belong to them. I believe that just the existence of this fact had its own painful psychological repetition for generations. I think we want to forget all the hatred, grief, and pain of the American slavery plantation system. It can be too much to think on—even now. However, it is a past that will not go away without the allowance of the truth of those slavery times.

> Master Teed Sharpe, Jr. had said he was going to make my brother Peter do as much work as my sister did. She was a young girl, but grown, and stout, and strong. Peter couldn't keep up with her. He wasn't old enough nor strong enough, then. He would have been later, but he hadn't reached his growth and my sister had. Every time that Peter would fall behind my sister, Teed would take him out and buckle him down to a log with a leather strap, and stand way back and then he would lay that long cowhide down, up and down his back. He would split open with every stroke, and the blood would run down. The last time he turned Peter lose, Peter went to my sister and asked her for a rag. She thought he just wanted to wipe the blood out of his face and eyes, but when she gave it to him, he fell down dead across the potato ridges.
>
> *Robert Farmer, former slave (Cited in Mellon, 1988, p. 239)*

In my own Southern upbringing, I remember my parents speaking about the direct effects of slavery on us as a 20th-century family.

This is probably related to the fact that we still lived in Georgetown, a small Southern town that was once a way-station port for producing and shipping rice up and down the Waccamaw River. The town, founded in 1729, was a port (1732), for the delivery of slaves and the local area was a continuance of plantations that contributed to the breeding of slave children. Charleston and Georgetown, South Carolina, and the surrounding plantations were the birth locations of many of my ancestors. Large British family plantations developed in the area in the early 18th century. After the American Revolution, the plantation system was continued by their British descendants. These plantations of cotton and rice thrived on black slave labor into the 19th century, up until the Civil War and even beyond that war:

> Africans and their descendants had been cultivating rice on the Waccamaw since the eighteenth century, clearing the swamps and marshlands to create the great plantations, digging and ditching, building the banks to hold back the waters when not desired .... "All dem rice field been nothing but swamp.

Slavery people cut kennel (canal) and cut down woods—and dig ditch through raw woods. All been clear up for plant rice by slavery people."

(Joyner, 1984, p. 42)

I sometimes wondered why my parents and I never had more conversations regarding slavery. Was it too painful to recount and continue to live on the earth that so many of us had died on in service to the plantation system? My parents oftentimes made reference to the contemporary racial bias and prejudice that they experienced at first hand living as children and later adults in a small Southern town. They spoke with one another, infrequently with me, about these things. My mother and father spoke about "slavery time," from what they had heard from their own parents, and grandparents.

I know they must have had phantom *memory*, an archetypal presence within them that had been there since even before our ancestors were enslaved. I believe that they knew things about slavery that they never brought fully into consciousness from the stored unconscious memories of their grandparents, and therefore could not share with me. I know this because my grandparents spoke about their grandparents and aunts who themselves had worked on cotton plantations.

I think it can be the not telling of the historical slave narrative that truly still haunts us—both whites and blacks. Our American history has glazed over many such stories, thus supporting a collective amnesia that has only benefited the continuation of racism in our society. We as Americans could only be desirous of creating a narrative of amnesia that denies the pain of American slavery. The details have been "made" coincidental. This is both an intentional and unconscious elimination of the details of the facts of slavery as in the manner in which complexes—even racial complexes can cause us to forget.

The truth for many African Americans is that even though we do not know the exact facts of slavery, we know in our archetypal bodies, energies and consciousness all that the history books and literature have failed to tell. Slavery's anguish, barely imaginable, continues to live with the ego observer us as we watch contemporary events, and also within some unconscious part of ourselves, remembering the brutality with which we saw ourselves live through and after slavery in ancestral, phantom memory. These cultural historical moments haunt us.

Archetypal Grief: Slavery's Legacy of Intergeneration Child Loss brings those moments that may have belonged only to mothering slaves and their children into a moment of conscious remembrance that recalls ancestral suffering, and honors their resilience, strength and spirit.

1
ARCHETYPES OF THE COLLECTIVE UNCONSCIOUS

The collective unconscious

Archetypes were defined by Jung as forms or patterns as well as an energy force that exist within human consciousness and therefore throughout the human experience, during the time of our existence. In the writing of his book *The Archetypes and the Collective Unconscious*, ([1959] 1980) Jung felt that he established the idea of an unconscious that had been in development for decades through the work of Freud and others before him. The idea of an archetype had presented itself to Plato centuries ago. In his investigation of the unconscious mind Jung furthered his work by naming the concept of archetypes. From 1933 onward Jung began writing about the unconscious and the archetypes. In describing the unconscious Jung states:

> A more or less superficial layer of the unconscious is undoubtedly personal. I call it the personal unconscious. But this *personal unconscious* rests upon a deeper layer, which does not derive from personal experience and is not a personal acquisition but is inborn. This deeper layer I call the *collective unconscious*. I have chosen the term "collective" because this part of the unconscious is not individual but universal.
>
> *(CW9i, para. 3; emphasis in the original)*

A most significant identification for Jung regarding the collective unconscious was that unlike Freud, Jung did not think of it as the place for only that which was hidden from the conscious ego, and capable of holding only repressed content. Jung believed that the unconscious held the possibilities for a richness that would complement the human ego. This richness included mythologies, dreams, telos and the potential for a deeper understanding of life's meaning. Jung believed that there was a separation of consciousness in humans, one side with personal unconscious material made up mostly of complexes. On the other side would have been the material of the collective unconscious consisting primarily of archetypes.

In speaking further of the collective unconscious Jung says:

> In contrast to the personal psyche, it has contents and modes of behavior that are more or less the same everywhere and in all individuals. It is, in other words, identical in all men and thus constitutes a common psychic substrate of a suprapersonal nature which is present in every one of us.
>
> (CW9i, para. 3)

It is important to note in the above quote that Jung recognizes that the contents and what he calls "modes of behavior" belong to *all men*. I would add *and all women*. I believe his intention was to be inclusive of women; however, with the sometimes mixed words that Jung used to describe women, and the more recent unveiling of gender biases not only on Jung's writing but also in that of other male writers, it seems important to indicate the explicit *inclusion* of women.

Jung states, "The archetype is essentially an unconscious content that is altered by becoming conscious and by being perceived, and it takes its colour from the individual consciousness in which it happens to appear" (CW9i, para. 6). In more recent times, we have come to recognize this color as the *cultural* aspect of the archetype showing itself. Jung was careful to examine many different cultures over many decades seeking to find the commonality in the archetypes that was the cause of a universal pattern. One of his major contributions was the recognition of this universal pattern in our mythologies.

Jung is specific about the characteristics of the archetypes, and as several Jungian thinkers have done over the years, he has provided the archetypes with clearly defined attributes. Jung first described such attributes in *Four Archetypes: Mother/Rebirth/Spirit/Trickster* (CW9i).

One of Jung's most important and descriptive analyses of an archetype was that of the Self. In *Memories, Dreams, Reflections,* Jung's autobiography, he details his initial encounter with his own archetypal Self through a dream:

> I found myself in a dirty, sooty city. It was night, and winter, and dark, and raining. I was in Liverpool. With a number of Swiss—say half a dozen. I walked through the dark streets. I had the feeling that there we were coming from the harbor, and that the real city was actually up above, on the cliffs. We climbed up there. It reminded me of Basel, where the market is down below and then you go up through the Totengasschen (Alley of the Dead), which leads to a plateau above and so to the Petersplatz and the Peterskirche.
>
> When we reached the plateau, we found a broad square dimly illuminated by street lights, into which many streets converged. The various quarters of the city were arranged radially around the square. In the center was a round pool, and in the middle of it a small island. While everything round about was

obscured by rain, fog, smoke and dimly lit darkness, the little island blazed with sunlight. On it stood a single tree, a magnolia, in a shower of reddish blossoms. It was as though the tree stood in the sunlight and were at the same time the source of light. My companions commented on the abominable weather, and obviously did not see the tree. They spoke of another Swiss who was living in Liverpool, and expressed surprise that he should have settled here. I was carried away by the beauty of the flowering tree and the sunlit island, and thought, "I know very well why he has settled here." Then I awoke.

(1973: pp. 197–198)

Jung says of the above dream that it clarified and defined for him all the previous work that he had completed both personally and professionally. He indicated that this dream spoke to his understanding of the center of the psyche, the unconscious as being the Self, and from this dream he was able to recognize this controlling center. Jung's idea regarding the significance of the Self archetype relates to his firm belief in his own "empirical" studies of the unconscious and archetypes.

The archetypes

Archetypal Grief: Slavery's Legacy of Intergenerational Child Loss introduces us to the archetypes through the language, images and behavior of those victims of slavery who share their stories. Jung states that the archetypes show themselves through our mythology and within the selective culture in which we happen to be born. The behavior of those in this particular case is usually the emotional psychological behavior of grief, mourning and sadness. It will also include anger. These narratives do not belong only to those who lived through slavery but also to those who have spent years thinking and writing about the individuals who witnessed and were a part of African Holocaust—slavery. In fact, these narratives belong to all of us. Contemporary narratives of the descendants living today, who I believe continue to experience the effects of slavery's legacy, also have the right to a voice in these pages. Perhaps it is important to define all the words in the book's title. The theme of the book may demand intimacy and close examination of each word of this title.

Jung's theoretical model of the personal and collective unconscious cannot be discussed without giving consideration to archetypes and *culture*—Africanist and Eurocentric. Samuel Kimbles in *Phantom Narratives: The Unseen Contributions of Culture to Psyche* says the following:

> I believe there is a group archetype that gets expressed through cultural complex constellations, which are as active in societal contexts at large as they are in our institutional life. This means that analysts' and patients' cultural histories, as well as the emergence and functioning of analysis are structured by archetypal dynamics.

(2014, p. 110)

When Jung introduced his archetypes, he provided a good deal of cultural attributes. These European models of culture have dominated Jungian psychology though there have been intermittent connections made to other cultures—yoga and Buddhism, for example. There has been minimal positive reference on Jung's part to Africanist cultural traditions to any great extent.

The archetypes inhabit our world as we inhabit theirs whether we think of them as patterns, energies, "real" gods or goddesses. These energies inform us about our other selves—not only of the ego, even if we believe that they are no long-lasting innate godly presences, but rather only parts of cognitive brain functioning or mental representatives. Our stories as humans, the mythologies of how we come to live as we do, Jung says have developed from these archetypes, living in psyche, acting through us as we work to become more conscious and conscientious. The results of the presence of archetypes take shape with a cultural mask. The cultural masks of the African diaspora who have followed the Yoruba religious tradition appear in the spiritual practices of Voudou, Christianity, as well as Santeria. In discussing Santeria and the Orisha, the author of *Santeria: The Religion*, Migene Gonzalez-Wippler says:

> Santeria is an earth religion, a magico-religious system that has its roots in nature and natural forces. Each orisha or saint is identified with a force of nature and with a human interest or endeavor …. Oshun symbolizes river waters but is also the patron of love and marriage, fertility, and gold. She is essentially the archetype of joy and pleasure. Yemaya is identified with the sea but is also the symbol of motherhood and protects women in their endeavors.
> *(1989, p. 4)*

Archetypal grief within the context of this writing has to do with a particular type of grief and mourning. I use the word archetypal to signify the long-standing existence of an emotional state related to the energy of archetypes and patterned in a particular form that becomes recognizable in a given cultural environment. This behavior of grief is not just present for a few hours or days.

Rather, I am suggesting that because of the traumatic nature and longevity of this type of grief, due to centuries of American slavery—cultural trauma—it has become powerful and reflective of centuries-long archetypal *potentiality* that becomes active at a cross-generational level. Furthermore, I am suggesting that this *potentiality* becomes realized in the behavior and lived experiences of people of color. The historical presence of slavery and its profound effect on African Americans has supported the development of a psychic state showing itself as an *ever-present grief* through generations.

One characteristic of this archetypal grief is that it is selective—it has surrounded and presented itself to a particular group of women, those women of color—mothering slaves—who have given birth to children, and also those who have not, because the mother archetype is still always available to women who do not participate in becoming pregnant. In this selectivity, the relatedness of suffering connected to slavery and its post-Reconstruction realism is still present in contemporary times. African American women display a particular type of depression, sadness and anticipatory fear directly related to their children. This sadness precludes any conscious idea that they do not want their children to do well. African American women *must* take on the mantle of savior for their children. This aspect of the mother—birth mother driven by an emotional complex, or by the mother archetype—can be there for any mother. It can be constellated by the cultural complex in the form of protection—some might think overprotection. A cloak of protection for Africanist children is in part due to the legacy of need based on the psychological persecution of African American children since slavery.

It began with their control and threatened removal from their parents at the will of slave owners causing great potential anxiety in enslaved children. It continued in the violence these children had to witness or receive as slaves.

Archetypes, neuroscience and epigenetics

Our view of archetypal psychology has been shifting and changing minimally since Jung first introduced his concept of the archetypes. He could be unclear in his own definitions as related to the location and biology of the archetypes. In following his lead, many Jungians have a view of archetypes as psycho-spiritual entities. There is an acknowledgement in this perspective that archetypes are both a type of energy as well as a pattern—a mode. It is a force that creates a certain type of consciousness by taking shape within the mind/being of humans. This shape-taking ability will conform to the individual (including culture), having an experience of the archetype. Each society will display the archetypal energy and forces in individuals as well as collective groups. The location of these archetypes remains in human consciousness in a way that holds us yet where we are unable to have direct knowledge of their location or an explanation of how they come to and through us. Jung defines them as being a part of our DNA.

They are a great part of what makes us divine. Early references to the archetypes suggest that they are spiritual entities—gods and goddesses, mythological figures that possess emotional tones, psychic attributes that come into human awareness.

The above has been an accepted classical Jungian view of the archetypes for a long time. Other references to the archetypes relate to their imagery making. In *Complex Archetype Symbol*, Jolande Jacobi says: "By 'primordial images' Jung then meant all the mythologems, all the legendary or fairy-tale motifs, etc. which concentrate universally modes of behavior into images, or perceptible patterns" (1959, p. 33).

In more recent times new scientific explorations into human brain functioning suggests that there is a biological underpinning for the continuation of what Jung called an archetypal DNA in human consciousness and the collective unconscious. The idea of an internal mental model has been considered by the Jungian analyst, Jean Knox. In *Archetype, Attachment, Analysis: Jungian Psychology and the Emergent Mind*, Knox draws on her understanding of archetypes:

Research, much of it within an attachment theory framework, demonstrates that our expectations of the world are governed not by rules of formal logic but by implicit and explicit mental models which organize and give a pattern to our experience. The archetype, as image schema, provides an initial scaffolding for this process, but the content is provided by real experience, particularly that of intense relationships with parents and other key attachment figures stored in the form of internal working models in implicit memory.

(2012, p. 9)

Knox brings to the discussion her ideas regarding attachment theory and cognitive science views on archetypes. In discussing Jung, Knox says:

Although Jung fully acknowledged the crucial role that personal experience plays in the formation of the unconscious internal world he struggled in his attempt to provide an integrated account of the interaction of real experience with innate psychic content and he did not offer any significant discussion of psychological development in infancy and childhood.

(Ibid., p. 88)

Recent studies in neuroscience indicate that one avenue of "real experience" could be caused by *mirror neurons* researched by Giacomo Rizzolatti in his study of monkeys in 1992. Rizzolatti and a group of scientists were completing research on the motor function of monkeys. During their study of that part of the monkey's brain known as F5, they noticed that in a hand-grasping exercise, one monkey observing the movement of another responded in an imitative motor pattern mimicking the pattern of the first monkey. The scientists initially believed that this was an error but as they repeated the experiments, they discovered that the brain function of "imitation" occurred in the brain cells of the observing monkey following the pattern of action in the watched monkey. Rizzolatti discovered over time that the mere suggestion that a future action would occur caused motor neuron cells to fire in at first monkeys, and later in humans during the course of experiments between subject and observers.

An accompanying fact as explained by Rizzolatti and Corrado Sinigaglia in *Mirrors in the Brain: How Our Minds Share Actions and Emotion*, recognizes that though we can perform an imitative behavior, we may not have intentionality or an understanding of this behavior. In the chapter on "Imitation and Language", the authors note:

This is not to say that the presence of a mirror neuron system, such as that found in monkeys, is sufficient to explain the emergence of intentional, or even linguistic, communicative behavior. We have seen this when talking about imitation: it is one thing to understand an action, quite another to imitate an action we have observed.

(2008, p. 153)

It may appear far afield to think about mirror neurons in view of this writing regarding archetypes and an emotive archetypal experience such as grief. It may even seem contradictory. However, when I consider the structure of the human brain, cognitive sciences and what has been discovered in the last twenty years regarding brain functioning and environmental influences, the idea of an archetypal influence does not appear remote or impossible. This is partly due to the definition of that which is archetypal—being an original pattern in which we can as human beings fill and alter. What might be the relationship between the development of long-standing archetypal grief, (fitting into a pattern of human suffering), on the development of brain functioning in women under centuries-long trauma circumstances? Does the brain change? How? I believe that it is valuable to pose questions regarding the inter-relationship between the longevity of an archetypal emotion such as grief—it is just as long-standing in our human experiences as pain, and the connection to its influence over cellular brain structure open to change, by environmental factors.

I would suggest that the relationship between the two—human brain cells biology in production of imitated behavior of one another could be an important aspect of intergenerational trauma and accompanying what I have termed archetypal grief. Did American slavery create a change in the archetypal patterning of women of color that would manifest itself in an intergenerational patterning of emotion—grief?

How likely is it that over a period of time—in our case centuries of slavery—might it be that daughter following mother following daughter in a line of girls and women bred to be slaves, could acquire and develop in neurological as well as psychological interconnected patterns, an experience of grief. This grief is learned through the interaction of maternal behaviors of mothering slaves and the characteristics of American slavery. Jung has stated:

> It is a mistake to suppose that the psyche of the newborn child is a tabula rasa in the sense that there is absolutely nothing in it. In so far as the child is born with a differentiated brain that is predetermined by heredity and therefore individualized, it meets sensory stimuli coming from outside, not with any aptitudes but with specific ones .... These aptitudes can be shown to be inherited instincts and preformed patterns, the latter being the *a priori* and formal conditions of apperception that are based on instinct.
> *(CW9i, para. 136)*

2
THE MOTHER ARCHETYPE

Orisha bi iya kosi
Iya la ba ma a bo

There is no deity like mother
It is the mother that is worthy
Of being worshipped

Nigerian proverb

Goddess and mother attachment

> In worshipping her as "She Who Weeps," the ancient Egyptians acknowledged Isis as the source of their prosperity, the Maternal and the source of their lives. Herodotus has recorded, "Egypt is the gift of the Nile." The Egyptians believed that the Nile began with Isis' tears splashing from the heavens as she mourned her murdered husband/son Osiris.
>
> *(Sertima, 1997, p. 64)*

The mother archetype was one of the first parts of the collected unconscious to be written about by Jung. This of course makes sense since the mother brings children into the world and is regarded as the source of creation and continued life. Mythologies from around the world tell of woman as creator of human life. Jung says the following regarding the mother archetype:

> Like any other archetype, the mother archetype appears under an almost infinite variety of aspects. I mention here only some of the more characteristic. First in importance are the personal mother and grandmother, stepmother and mother-in-law; then any woman with whom a relationship exists—for

example, a nurse or governess or perhaps a remote ancestress. Then there are what might be termed mothers in a figurative sense. To this category belongs the goddess, and especially the Mother of God, the Virgin, and Sophia.

(CW9i, para. 156)

The image of Isis weeping is a mythological one that helps to establish a Mother of Sorrow archetype. From this archetypal maternal lineage we are able to find other instances—the mother of Moses who set her son adrift down the Nile River, and Mary mother of Jesus, holding her crucified son. To the images of this particular archetype we can add that of Yemoja who traveled to the Americas with the African diaspora.

In a further discussion of the mother archetype Jung states:

> My own view differs from that of other medico-psychological theories principally in that I attribute to the personal mother only a limited aetiological significance. This is to say, all those influences which the literature describes as being exerted on the children do not come from the mother herself, but rather from the archetype projected upon her, which gives her a mythological background and invests her with authority and numinosity.
>
> *(CW9i, para. 159)*

In the *African Unconscious: Roots of Ancient Mysticism and Modern Psychology*, Edward Bruce Bynum addresses the presence of an unconscious of which archetypes are composed. In his definition of the unconscious mind, Bynam states:

> Generally speaking, it means a dimension of mental life in which information is processed outside of conscious awareness. The recognition of this arches back to the ancient Kemetic idea of the creative flux out of which life and conscious awareness arises, the so-called Primeval Waters of Nun.
>
> *(Bynum, 2012, p. 81)*

The idea that there is a "place" of "non-locality" which belongs to a deeper consciousness when "discovered" was brought into modern thought first through the work of Freud, and later Jung. The history of the unconscious has been, according to Bynum, conceived to be present and accessible for centuries before both Jung and Freud.

> All the hominid variations, from the early and primitive lost Pre-Australopithecines, to the Australopithecines we know of, to Homo habilis to Homo erectus and eventually to Homo sapiens, unfolded on the same continent shaped like a skull looking eastward on the planet .... Their deep recurrent experiences, their racial memories are rooted in our own brains in a collective, primordial way.
>
> *(Ibid., p. 78)*

Bynum notes that Freud referred to the collective unconscious as the "racial memory" (ibid.). There has been more discussion, and equally less agreement, about what archetypes actually are over the years. Do they really exist as Jean Knox has questioned as "metaphysical entities which are eternal and therefore independent of the body" in her discussion of one of what she believes to be Jung's definitions of archetypes (Knox, 2012, p. 60) This appears to be a belief of many who do not relinquish the idea that archetypes can be without a specific bodily location and yet can come into conscious awareness. The possibility that we can be "possessed" by an archetypal energy that make us unaware of our conscious behaviors until further integration by "ego work" is a familiar element of classical Jungian psychoanalysis. Is it outdated to hold onto such classical Jungian thinking regarding archetypes? Are we to hold onto the following as Jacobi has stated:

> Like a seed the psyche bears within it the predisposition to full maturity and realizes this predisposition in the form of archetypal processes …. And since all psychic life is absolutely grounded in archetypes, and since we can speak not only of archetypes, but equally well of archetypal situations, experiences, actions, feelings, insights, etc., any hidebound limitation of the concept would only detract from its richness of meaning and implication.
>
> *([1959] 1971, p. 59)*

My proposition that there is such an "archetypal situation"—feelings as archetypal grief—does not seek to challenge the theories of others who take a defining stance of archetypes as image schema, mirrored neurons or from a spiritual-mystical tradition. I would like to propose that since the beginning of the development of Jung's multi-sided view of the archetype, we are able to choose our belief system based not only on current neuroscience beliefs but also on a personally held spiritual orientation. It would appear that the idea of a mother archetype has great merit because of all the mythology, images and psychological importance of *mother* through the history of humankind. This certainly includes the spiritual. Perhaps Jung was able to be so varied in his own writing about the archetypes because he could be expansive concerning his belief in our biological selves and he even referenced the possible future of this topic as important to our understanding of archetypes. In choosing to believe in the existence of an innate unconscious self, influenced by an internal physiological system dependent upon a particular environment, I would propose that all three of these elements can co-exist together. One does not necessarily disprove the other but only adds to our contemporary knowledge of what is possible for us as human beings in the realm of consciousness.

Jung's work in the area of psychology included his research into many other areas of human endeavors including mythology, alchemy and religion. These important areas of his study proved to be inclusive of and referential to his belief in the existence of a collective unconscious. The unconscious that holds the pattern of the mother archetype allows for the bringing forth of that which belongs to the personal mother, in Jung's terminology. He states:

I myself make it a rule to look first for the cause of infantile neuroses in the mother, as I know from experience that a child is much more likely to develop normally than neurotically, and that in the great majority of cases definite causes of disturbances can be found in the parents, especially in the mother.

(CW9i, para. 159)

We can see that Jung believes that the personality of the mother plays a larger part in the development of the child. Though Jung is not considered to be an important spokesperson for child development, we can see from the above statement that he has sufficient knowledge to recognize the emotional and psychological influence of a mother on her child. He further suggests that the child projects archetypally onto the mother. Later, Michael Fordham in his own study of infants and their mothers, entitled *Abandonment in Infancy*, found that this is an unlikely experience of an infant (1985, p. 19). However, by the time the child under observation was ten weeks old, there were indications of behavior that Fordham saw as archetypal:

I regard N's experience as archetypal but without much mental imagery. One is reminded of Jung's metaphor (1969b) of the spectrum, in which archetypal experience took on many forms. At the infrared end, the experiences merged into physical action. It is to this end that we have to look in order to understand what happened.

(Ibid.)

The idea of the existence of a force, an energy that holds the human experience within itself, and makes itself known to our awareness at times through conscious acts, is inclusive of the possibility of an archetypal situation such as grief. This emotional state of grief that passes through generations of African American and other women of color who have lost children to traumatic events, I believe, can be examined from a holistic view of the numinous aspect of the mother archetype as well as the personal-physiological elements of neurobiology.

There is the possibility that over time that which initially showed itself as archetypal became more influential as a factor of epigenetics due to the conditions of slavery. What might be the relationship between these two forces? What does it take to learn about, know and accept the influences of slavery on birthing mothers' psyches? What could be the influence of archetypal mother-goddess energy?

African mythology within an African American context

I believe that there are several threads of spiritual practice operative among African Americans. In the last twenty-five years, many more individuals have actively sought a closer identity and involvement with African-oriented spiritual practices. These include practitioners of Santeria and Voudou. Others continue in the Protestant religion of their family and African American ancestors. Women such as

Harriet Tubman and Sojourner Truth converted to Protestantism but appeared to speak with the spirit of the Orisha. There is a questioning unrest regarding traditional Protestantism among African Americans that is reflected in loss of membership in the traditional church by those seeking a more "charismatic" or neo-Pentecostal interpretation of their faith. In *The Black Church in the African American Experience* (1990), Lincoln and Mamiya define this loss of membership in their chapter entitled "Challenges to the Black Church." Factors influencing the decline include African American men who chose to become Muslim and follow the Islamic religion. A lack of church growth is attributed to the absence of young adults, primarily male, without church affiliation—the *unchurched*.

A third factor is the current political and economic climate in America, which began to provide support typically given within the African American church. As professional African Americans move into the middle class, the church is viewed as less of an economic, social and political necessity than in former times. I have not seen studies that draw correlations between levels of discontent and a lack of connection based on spiritual lineage, but am curious about this possibility.

Henry Louis Gates, Jr., in *The Signifying Monkey* (1988), explored Esu (or Legba), a mythological god from the Yoruba tradition. Gates defined mythology using Esu as a model. He stated that Africans did not arrive in America with a *tabula rasa* ("blank slate") but with the cultures of their heritage. Esu's survival in the New World is evidence of this transport of culture.

Gates described Esu as messenger of the gods. Like Hermes, the Greek messenger god, Esu traveled between the gods and humans, living between two worlds. In this way, Esu survived in countless mythologies, serving not only as messenger but also as trickster god, creating chaos and confusion. In his more spiritual function, Esu was able to "read the signs" of Ifa divination as taught to him by Ifa. Esu served as divine interpreter of the Ifa oracle, interpreting it to humankind on behalf of the gods.

Esu, who was sometimes known as Legba, acquired a monkey as a companion when brought to the Americas during the time of slavery. This monkey appeared to have become the possessor of the "tricks" for which Esu was known in Africa. Esu was known for his duality. He was distinguished among the Yoruba gods for creating chaos and confusion, and for returning during the most passionate, embittered exchange to offer a rational, calming solution to a problem he himself had created. Esu was both male and female. He was an unknown factor, and always created uncertainty whenever he traveled among humans.

One of his greatest powers was his ability to connect with and interpret life's events. According to Yoruba tradition, just before birth we are given knowledge through our *ori* (head) of who we are to become. We choose the life we live. At birth we forget these choices, and Ifa divination serves to help us to remember our destiny. Esu was the mythological god who served as mediator in this spiritual task. As one seeks understanding and interpretation of myth, Gates (1988) suggested that it is through Esu that one can expect to find answers as well as divine knowledge.

African Americans have a spiritual tradition that is strong, even though traditional African slave spiritual practices were forbidden by slaveholders. These culturally different practices were held to be demonic or heathen. In accommodating themselves to their new environment, these first American Africans incorporated the slaveholders' Christian religious beliefs into their own. Today, in different parts of North America, there exist communities of Ifa, a Yoruba religion of Nigeria. In Ifa, divination continues as a spiritual practice as it has for centuries. The *babalow* (spiritual priest of Ifa) assisted by Esu and others of the Orisha, provide spiritual direction. This African religion has maintained the character of its African origin without much influence from European religion. Other religions of Africanist people such as Baptist, Pentecostal and African Methodist Episcopal more clearly show this influence.

If it is true that we bring forward our ancestral/archetypal patterns, how might they show themselves in today's religious practices? Santeria is practiced mostly among South Americans and Cubans. What of the integrative spiritual practices of African Americans? What form do they take? How might they evolve archetypally?

African goddess: Yemoja

In *The Way of the Orisha*, Philip John Neimark gives us this definition of Ifa:

> The philosophy of Ifa originated with the Yoruba peoples of West Africa in what is now Nigeria. Ifa mythology relates that the creation of humankind arose in the sacred city of Ile Ife just outside what is now Lagos. The Yoruba created a highly sophisticated city-state empire, which according to many anthropologists, was on a par with that of ancient Athens. Their philosophy reflected an integration of the basic truths and wisdom of nature with the equally true, but vastly different, demands of a sophisticated commercial culture. Ifa was not a product of superstition, ignorance, or lack of education but years of practice and refinement by successful, intelligent, and highly educated men and women who used it for the simplest of reasons: it worked!
>
> *(1993, p. 13)*

In the Yoruba tradition Yemoja/Yemaya is known as the Mother of the Ocean as well as the mother of all the Yoruba deities and the goddess of fertility. Yemoja is the goddess who protects mothers and watches over children. Because she is the mother goddess she takes care of children in the absence of Oshun, the Nigerian goddess of beauty. One of the ironies of the sacred trust of Yemoja is that she is also known as the protector of sailors. As slave ship crews crossed the Atlantic Ocean with their human cargos of Africanist people, it is likely that early African slaves were imploring Yemoja for release from the slave ship hold.

The African goddess Yemoja is only one of many who made their travels to South and North America as archetypes under the cover of Catholicism. Slaves traveling to South and North America, Cuba and Haiti brought Yemoja as their archetypal mother who later became the Virgin Mary.

Attachment

In traditional African society the relationship between being human and being with the divine is believed to have originated before birth. This is partially true due to a belief in reincarnation, and also due to the connection between Africans and the community engagement with spirituality, as practiced within a model that recognizes and honors rituals connected with a particular god or goddess. Even with the emergence in Africa of other religions such as Islam and Christianity centuries ago, the traditional spiritual practices continue. The underlying beliefs of these traditional practices support an attachment not only to a recognition of an ancestral lineage that is unbroken but also to an attachment at a conscious level to the mother-child bond. The close tie of respect for this bond is an aspect of cultural life. This can be seen in the rituals following the birth of children. These post-birth rituals are described by John Mbiti in *African Religion and Philosophy*:

> The placenta and umbilical cord are the symbols of the child's attachment to mother, to womanhood, to the state of inactivity. They are therefore the object of special treatment in most African societies. For example, the Gikuyu deposit the placenta in an uncultivated field and cover it with grain and grass, these symbolizing fertility. The uncultivated field is the symbol of fertility, strength and freshness; and using it is like a silent prayer that the mother's womb should remain fertile and strong for the birth of more children. Among the Didinga, the placenta is buried hear the house where the birth takes place; among the Ingassana it is put into a calabash which is hung on a special tree (*gammeiza*); and among the Wolof the placenta is buried in the back-yard, but the umbilical cord is sometimes made into a charm which the child is made to wear.
>
> *(1989, pp. 109–110)*

When describing early African American childbirth customs, Melville Herskovits says in his chapter entitled "Africanisms in Secular Life" that "The care used in disposing of the placenta and the treatment of the navel cord are also largely African" (1958, p. 189). This would indicate to me that such childbirth rituals which were accompanied by care of the placenta and what it represents—fertility, sacredness and continuity of life—were preserved for a time in African diaspora life. The significance of the physical attachment between mother and child underscores the psychological connection.

The work of John Bowlby and his attachment theory has greatly influenced our clinical understanding of how children develop a bond with their mothers and surrogates and how they experience stress when this bonding does not occur in a healthy way. In his trilogy *Attachment and Loss* (1980) Bowlby provides detailed studies—his own and that of other child researchers—that explore children's anxiety, anger, sadness, depression, attachment and loss in relation to their primary caretakers. The childhood loss of enslaved children has its own markers different from even those of foster or abandoned children, even though some features remain the same. The unique features of enslavement carries its own branding. The following narrative is from *We Are Your Sisters: Black Women in the Nineteenth Century*, edited by Dorothy Sterling:

> Interviewed after the war, Harriet Tubman, the legendary Underground Railroad conductor, described the first time she ran away.
>
> I was only seven years old when I was sent away to take car' of a baby. One mornin' after breakfast I stood by de table waitin' till I was to take it; just by me was a bowl of lumps of white sugar. Now you know, Missus, I never had nothing good; no sweet, no sugar, an dat sugar, right by me, did look so nice, an' Missus's back was turned to me so I jes' put my fingers in de sugar bowl to take one lump, an' she turned an saw me.
>
> De nex' minute she had de raw hide down; I give one jump out of de do', an' I see dey came after me, but I just' flew, and dey did't catch me. I run, an I run, an I run.
>
> By an by when I was clar tuckered out, I come to a great big pig-pen. Dar was an ole sow dar, an' perhaps eight or ten little pigs. I was too litte to climb into it, but I tumbled ober de high board, an fell in on de ground; I was so beat out I couln't stir.... An' dere Missus, I stayed from Friday till de nex' Chuesday, fightin' wid dose little pigs for de potato peelin's an' oder scraps dat came down in de trough. De old sow would push me away when I tried to git her chillen's food, an I was awful afread of her. By Chuesday I was so starved I knowed I'd got to go back to my Missus, I hadn't got no whar else to go.
>
> *(1984, pp. 9–10)*

This childhood experience from a woman who was to become a representative of the *archetype of freedom* was not uncommon for enslaved Africanist children. The exceptional life of enslaved children imprinted on them the mark of those who had seen the worst violence of human nature, though from most reports this image of violence could be accompanied by a laissez-faire approach by whites which provided a somewhat cocooned childhood. Later in this book I will discuss the nature of this "protected" childhood for African American children. Like all situations that involved slavery, the childhood of these children was secure, but certainly not in the way that Bowlby has described in his own writings. The security of the children depended almost solely on the power, personality and type of intervention of the slave owner—modeling through words or behavior—whippings or death. The attachment between mother and child was tenuous at best depending on the psychology of the plantation owner to whom they were enslaved. History shows us that owners could be cruel or make attempts to show "kindness" towards enslaved Africanist people—or they could simply be psychopaths. The underlying factor which can be forgotten by some who tell slavery's story is that African Americans were enslaved and *should not have been*.

It does not matter what kind of treatment they received at the hands of slave owners. Their lives in bondage was against human laws of compassion. It appears that many African American children spent their childhoods before the age of eight or ten free to play with their black peers, under the care of mother surrogates and sometimes their own mothers—though the latter was not guaranteed due to the demand for young women to work in the plantation fields. Most young children, watched over by grandmothers or elder black women during the day, were free to spend time playing with black and white children on the plantation.

Prior to the early days of infancy for black children, their womb experiences were sometimes protected and made safe by a slave owner who, valuing the pregnancy for what was offered economically, allowed the enslaved mother to have a more "easy" time of work on the plantation. However, the opposite was equally possible. Black women were usually required to work right up until the birth of their children. Sometimes this work involved labor in the fields where they actually delivered their children, or in a quite different work environment. "In some cases women, anywhere from five to nine months pregnant, were put to work sewing, weaving, or spinning in the company of elderly, pregnant, or nursing women" (White, 1998, p. 110)

We now know that the emotional and psychological state of the mother directly effects the physical and emotional state of the child. I wonder not only about the children of enslaved mother after being birthed but also about their state when held in the mother's womb as she continued working. What of the condition of these children who would later become mothers themselves? What was the intergenerational trauma that their mothers received? What was passed on to them even when their early childhood was one of mostly play, thus shielding the visibility of most of the injustices of slavery that was to follow?

Bowlby's attachment theory includes a discussion of the anxiety and hostility of children. Many accounts of former slaves share the sadness not only of the children but also of their mothers. It seems rare to find instances of hostility towards the mothers. Perhaps this is a side of the formerly enslaved story that could not be revealed. How difficult it would be for an enslaved child to witness the stress of his/her enslaved mother and to add to this stress his/her own anger. It is unlikely that we could have an absolutely clear view into all the anxiety of formerly enslaved children; however, since the slavery era we have learned about Post Traumatic Stress Syndrome and the effects of experiencing stress and witnessing violence on children.

> The reason that anxiety about and hostility towards an attachment figure are so habitually found together, it is therefore concluded, is because both types of response are aroused by the same class of situation; and to a lesser degree, because, once intensely aroused, each response tends to aggravate the other. As a result, following experiences of repeated separation or threats of separation, it is common for a person to develop intensely anxious and possessive attachment behavior simultaneously with bitter anger directed against the

attachment figure, and often to combine both with much anxious concern about the safety of the figure.

(Bowlby, 1973, p. 256)

Separation: anxiety and anger

As I look at major theories of childhood developed by studies on culturally different children I find that there is no consideration of the area of my focus—cultural factors in descendant children of mothering slaves. I ask questions that pertain to an Africanist culture that endured intergenerational trauma. I can find very few, if any, references in the classical texts. This leads me to further believe that we must reimage ancestral and culture complexes, not by negating one's own cultural complex but by investigating the work with this complex invited as an essential aspect of exploration.

Only a few studies of enslaved mothers and their children have been carried out. I do not claim to have exclusive answers about this group of specially defined individuals. I do, however, claim that my interests lead me to them partially because their lives are a part of my cultural inheritance. This collective cultural inheritance including the trauma has oftentimes been made invisible, yet it deserves to be recognized, seen and claimed free from projected American collective shame.

3
RITES OF PASSAGE
Life and death

Traditional African beliefs

The essential model of life in traditional African society was based on rites of passage and their accompanying rituals. Two of the most important of these rites was the passage into life and the eventual passage into death. These two passages were seen as being intricately woven together. The accompanying mourning and celebration for each new death and each birth were acknowledged as reflections of the continuous lives of ancestors entering and leaving the same space. The Beng people have a word—*wrugbe*—which translates as *spirit village*. This is the place where souls return after death and also the place from where the souls of children leave to enter earth-bound lives. Anthropologist Amy Gottlieb lived in Bengland, Cote d'Ivoire, West Africa, and studied the cultural aspects of the lives of infants, children and parenting. Her book, *The Afterlife Is Where We Come From: The Culture of Infancy in West Africa* (2004), records the spiritual beliefs of reincarnation and the Beng community's beliefs regarding infants. She found these beliefs to be radically different to her own American culturally held beliefs, especially during her own pregnancy and with the subsequent birth of her children.

I find it important to reference the work of Gottlieb because it shows in the 21st century the continuation of ideas and beliefs regarding the rite of passage of birth that have survived for centuries. African culture still clings to many of its rituals.

Gottlieb writes that part of the birth ritual among the Beng was hastening to get the umbilical cord to fall off of the newly born infant so as to create the power of strength for leaving the *wrugbe* or else the child might die soon after birth. This is the power of the spiritual belief in not only the rite of passage but also in the rituals that reflect this particular passage of birth into life.

Rites of passage are not insignificant. The relationship between these rites and their survival or loss to the African diaspora are important in defining group cultural identity as well as individual psychological and spiritual development. Within the Beng culture, children enter the world as spiritual beings. They come from a place of spirit and will return to this place upon death.

The life of Beng babies

It seems unusual in our modern times to think about the rite of passage within the context of our ancestors or spiritual beliefs. This is not to say that we do not have rituals—baby showers, christening and naming ceremonies—we have, however, most certainly lost the ingrained texture of birth rituals and beliefs that still flourish in communities such as the Beng.

Gottlieb states:

> In the Beng world, infants are believed to emerge not from a void before gaining life inside a woman's womb, but from a rich, social existence in a place that adults call *wrugbe*. How do the Beng conceive of this culturally imaged space that is so critical to their understanding of the human life cycle? Several Beng adults explained that wrugbe is dispersed among invisible neighborhoods in major cities in African and Europe .... Given the rural nature of traditional Beng society, the imputed urban nature of wrugbe implies an other world that is truly Other.
>
> *(2004, p. 80; italic in the original)*

The importance of the children not entering the world from a void is most relevant. Reincarnation finds a place in Beng philosophy and as in most African societies is defined most easily through the *wrugbe*. Even within our general American collective religious beliefs we do not have a place where children and those recently dead are thought to communicate with one another. In one of the narrations of a former slave, she remembers being told that she and all the other black children were birthed into the world by way of a buzzard eggs. How did this variation on the stork story first come to life? We do not know but even in its telling we find the thread of racism as white children were brought by the white stork—a positive image. Black children were not; instead, they were delivered (birthed) by something that consumes dead flesh.

Gottlieb says:

> Once someone dies, the nenenj, or soul, is transformed into a *wru*, or spirit. Yet when that person is reincarnated as someone else, the *wru* nevertheless continues to exist as an ancestor. The ideology posits a dual, rather than an either/or existence. Unlike the classical Aristotelian framework, which demands that an identity be either one thing or another but not both simultaneously, the Beng view allows that a being may exist simultaneously at two very different levels of reality—the one visible and earthly, the other invisible and ghostly.
>
> *(2004, p. 82; italic in the original)*

In her study of and life with the Beng Gottlieb states that she was committed to exploring the philosophy of reincarnation which underpinned the Beng relationship with their infants and the "day-to-day experiences of actual babies and those who take care of them." In African American life, it was not uncommon to report some relationship with the interconnecting world of spirits:

> Did I ever see a spirit? 'Spect I has, and I sho' have felt one more than once. 'Spect I was born wid a caul over my eyes. When de last quarter of de moon come in de seventh month of a seventh year, is de most time you see spirits. Lyin' out in de moon befo' daybreak, I's smelt, I's heard, I's seed, and I's felt Catherine's spirit in de moon shadows. I come nigh catchin' hold of her one night, as I woke up a-dreamin' 'bout her, but befo' I could set up, I hear her pass 'way through de treetops dat I was layin', dreamin' under.
>
> *(Jesse Williams, former slave; cited in Mellon, 1988, p. 92)*

Within Beng rituals is the importance of the elimination of the umbilical cord. The removal of the cord through the application of a herbal mixture helps the newly born child to leave the *wrugbe* and become embodied. It is believed that the longer the cord remains intact, the more the child will be tempted to return to the *wrugbe* because its spirit continues to live there. A celebration ensues when the cord falls off and two additional rituals are performed. The first is an enema given by the mother.

> Typically a few hours after the first enema, the newborn is the subject of a second major ritual. The maternal grandmother or another older woman makes a necklace from a savanna grass of the same name. This necklace will be worn night and day by the infant to encourage general health and growth until it eventually tears and falls off.
>
> *(Gottlieb, 2004, p. 84)*

A third ritual is performed upon infant girls involving the piercing of the ears once the umbilical cord falls off. Even after these rituals have been performed great protection is afforded to the infants because there is a belief that the spirits may want to have the children return to them in the *wrugbe*—amounting to what Gottlieb terms *spirit kidnapping*.

Infants are carefully watched over not only by their mothers and maternal family members but also by diviners who are invited by the mother to visit with the child.

> This can occur whether children appear to be sick (missing the wrugbe) or well. This is where diviners enter the picture, for these specialists are seen as intermediaries between the living and the ancestors, as well as between the living and the bush spirits.
>
> *(Gottlieb, 2004, p. 87)*

In African American culture it was believed that children were very susceptible to death and would return to the spirit world if they were not protected and made strong enough to survive in this one. The bridge between the embodied world and the spirit world was thought be open at all times. It was important for families to know the ways of protecting their children.

Death and the future

In *African Religions and Philosophy*, John S. Mbiti says:

> The point here is that for Africans, the whole of existence is a religious phenomenon; man is a deeply religious being living in a religious universe. Failure to realize and appreciate this starting point has led missionaries, anthropologists, colonial administrators and other foreign writers on African religions to misunderstand not only the religions as such but the peoples of Africa.
> *(1989, p. 15)*

Mbiti devotes a chapter of this text to his discussion of the concept of time noting that in Swahili there are two words—*Sasa* and *Zamani*, which are used and connected to both concepts of life and death. Sasa time encompasses the "now-period"—"immediacy, nearness and now-ness." Mbiti says that it "is the period of immediate concern for people" (1989, p. 20) The definition of Zamani includes that state of time "beyond which nothing can go. Zamani is the graveyard of time, the period of termination .... it is the final storehouse for all phenomena and events, the ocean of time in which everything becomes absorbed into a reality that is neither after nor before" (ibid., p. 22).

In defining death, Mbiti says "death is a process which removes a person gradually from the Sasa period to the Zamani. After the physical death, the individual continues to exist in the Sasa period and does not immediately disappear from it."

The concept of time within the African framework as Mbiti explains it incorporates the idea of reincarnation through family members, a continued *spirit* presence even after physical death, the appearance of those who have died to still-living family members and the understanding that there is a state of *personal immortality*.

Mbiti says:

> This personal immortality is externalized in the physical continuation of the individual through procreation .... from the point of view of the survivors, personal immortality is expressed or externalized in acts like respecting the departed, giving bits of food to them, pouring out libation and carrying out instructions given by them either while they lived or when they appear.
> *(1989, p. 25)*

The concept of a personal immortality which is extended through procreation is an indication of importance: first, of women as mothers; and second, as a means to keep intact the societal fibers that hold a community together through ritualistic beliefs. If we consider Mbiti's words: "Procreation is the absolute way of insuring that a person is not cut off from personal immortality" (ibid., p. 25), then we might understand the underlying suffering in a mothering slave producing children. The philosophical core belief lies in the vitality of becoming pregnant and a mother—as this is essential to society as well as to the spirit of those who have gone before. With the idea of time as a spiral-constant that is always returning—not the Western idea of the linear birth then death, and perhaps a heaven, hell or purgatory—rituals are necessary to strengthen the psychological and spiritual essence of the individual as well as the community.

Mbiti describes an African consciousness where space and time are joined. He notes that this is especially true as regards Africans and their desire to remain physically close to their land. He says:

> The land provides them with roots of existence (Sasa), as well as binding them mystically to their departed. People walk on the graves of their forefathers, and it is feared that anything separating them from these ties will bring disaster to family and community life.
>
> *(Ibid., p. 26)*

The slave trade brought disaster to generations of African families and to that of the African diaspora. An examination of the philosophy of religion and spirituality that determined and infused African life can add to a deeper understanding of the traumatic rupture caused by slavery. A main justification for the continuation of slavery was the absence of African philosophies that safeguarded the sacred ritualized African life. A result of this was the racial lie projected onto the African diaspora that they had no religion, no philosophy, no soul. It made the enslavement and genocide of Africans more possible. It is always important to remember this when thinking of why white history wishes to erase any evidence of Africanist knowledge, religion or culture. It is just as important to reiterate the existence of these aspects of African life, and later in the life of the African diaspora, because even today as we exist in the 21st-century racism, in the form of white supremacy, remains relentless in its desire to strip Africanist people of any positive attributes—socially, morally or culturally.

Slavery, rites and rituals

In her most recent book, *Freedom is a Constant Struggle: Ferguson, Palestine, and the Foundations of a Movement*, Angela Y. Davis states in response to the interviewer's question regarding the struggle for freedom:

> I would say that as our struggles mature, they produce new ideas, new issues, and new terrains on which we engage in the quest for freedom. Like Nelson Mandela, we must be willing to embrace the long walk toward freedom.
>
> *(2016, p. 11)*

These words help us to remember that the struggle for freedom—and all of its positive life potential is not over. I believe that it also reminds us of the history we embody as it relates to Africanist rites of passage and rituals. Due to the trauma of slavery, there was a disruption in the pattern of these rituals. This is not to say that they were totally eliminated. Given the importance of these two passages—birth and death—I believe it is impossible to do away with rituals of some kind in the collective. Though in the 20th century, I think that we as a collective have rushed more and more towards the light of youthfulness and directly away from the idea of death. An example of this has been the discovery and use of Botox. Though it has multiple uses, a highly popular use has been for the maintenance of youthful skin and a slowdown in the aging process. As plastic surgery and Botox becomes more popular, women and men engage in the application of both—sometimes to their detriment, including death. The popular statement that "sixty is the new forty," are the exact words to describe a collective consciousness that wishes to stop aging and postpone death. It reflects a societal wish to continue living without having to consider any rite of passage that suggests aging and dying.

This is not a new criticism of an American collective consciousness. It has certainly shown up in the desire to freeze the body for future use and can be seen in the scientific development of methods of preserving the body.

There is no surprise in saying that Africanist skin is different than white skin. Not only in the visuals of color but also in the general receptivity to color and tolerance of heat. One of the truthfulness of science as regards African Americans is an acknowledgement of this difference in how heat effects black skin as opposed to white. This is also an aspect of cultural differences. It is not racism. Within the context of noting this difference is the widely held belief that members of the African diaspora require skin care that is different from whites. This is true in the same way that we require different treatment of our hair. This is not a surprise but can be taken by some as an aspect of black cultural life that should be a secret. When we consider the physical differences—without the overlay of racism—we notice and accept these physical differences.

These apparent skin differences connect with an underlying attitude towards life and death among African Americans. In the same way that we are self-identified and externally identified by the collective, we also know our beliefs through the care and texture of our skin. African Americans through generations of slavery came to deeply reaffirm the ancestral belief in life hereafter. This is connected to how one lives. This belief is not the one of heaven or hell as the only locations for soul/life but rather one which recognizes a continuum, sasa time, *wrugbe*.

As the centuries-long intergenerational loss of physical life progressed I believe that African traditional belief in the uninterrupted continuum of life and death in the way of renewal, survived in the consciousness of the African diaspora.

In *The Myth of the Negro Past*, Melville J. Herskovits states:

> The principle that life must have a proper ending as well as a well-protected beginning is the fundamental reason for the great importance of the funeral in

all Negro societies. This results from several causes, among the most important being the widespread African belief in the power of the ancestors to affect the life of their descendants. The place of this belief in the total African world view is in keeping with its significance for the people. For the dead are everywhere regarded as close to the forces that govern the universe, and are believed to influence the well-being of their descendants who properly serve them.

(1990, p. 197)

In Africanist consciousness there is no emotional struggle to preserve the skin or to take care of it in such a way as if it will mean the permanent preservation of the physical body—of life itself. This goes against the philosophical understanding that life continues, whether in the body of a recently passed ancestor or one from a longer period of time. It might seem insignificant to think about the consciousness of how we perceive our skin but in the narrative of racial relations and racism in the American collective, *skin as culture* has been and continues to be vitally important. From a depth psychological point of view, it is not only the surface that requires attention but also that which lies underneath. In considering the "underneath" of the body and our desire to preserve it or release it through death, there are cultural considerations that are dependent upon traditional spiritual and philosophical beliefs.

Since Africans held philosophical beliefs regarding the continued existence of the life force energy—inter-generationally—it would follow that the attention is not given to a singular bodily existence but rather by a perspective that incorporated a view of eternity through ancestors.

Herskovits says, "The ancestral cult resolves itself into a few essentials—the importance of the funeral, the need to assure the benevolence of the dead, and, in order to implement these points, concern with descent and kinship" (1958, p. 198) Plantation life for slaves held a constant view towards the possibility and likelihood of death—equally as much as birthing and life. These were of utmost significance because of the focused purpose of the plantation. The physical existence of slaves mattered immensely while at the same time their lives were considered insignificant to the owners of these plantations. The erratic, humiliating and murderous manner in which slaves were treated testified to both of these ways of being imprisoned. Slaves knew the truth of their circumstances. They were needed for the very survival of the plantations, yet their lives mattered little except for this survival of the economics of land.

David Brion Davis, in *Inhuman Bondage: The Rise and Fall of Slavery in the New World*, says:

As the Quaker John Woolman pointed out in the mid-eighteenth century, no human is saintly enough to be entrusted with total power over another. The slave was an inviting target for the hidden anger, passion, frustration, and revenge from which no human is exempt. A slave's work, leisure, movement, and daily fate depended on the largely unrestrained will of another person.

(2006, p. 198)

Would this have been part of the slave's psychological grief? How might this have added to their questioning of what life might have been like had they not been captured and imprisoned? What has happened or might happen to the continuum of ancestors and the slave's beliefs in a spiritual lineage beyond the physical body? Perhaps these questions can partially be answered too by the knowledge that Africans came to America and gave their rites of passage and rituals to the diaspora.

The essence of this connection allowed Africanist archetypal patterns to continue as potentiality in the lives of African Americans, showing itself in the culture. In *The Myth of the Negro Past*, Herskovits says:

> In West Africa, the ceremonial richness of the ancestral cult is enhanced because of the greater resources of the tribes of this region when compared to other areas, yet the feeling of the ever-present care afforded by these relatives in the world of the spirit is essentially the same among all African folk.
>
> *(1958, p. 198)*

This "sameness" was evident in the continued Africanist funeral rites among African Americans. The following is a description given by Herskovits which he says describes the slave African American funeral as reported by the author and anthropologist Newbell Puckett:

> There was one thing which the Negro greatly insisted upon, and which not even the most hard-hearted masters were ever quite willing to deny them. They could never bear that their dead could be put away without a funeral. Not that they expected, at the time of burial, to have the funeral service. Indeed, they did not desire it, and it was never according to their notions. A funeral to them was a pageant. It was a thing to be arranged for a long time ahead. It was to be marked by the gathering of kindred and friends from far and near. It was not satisfactory unless there was a vast and excitable crowd. It usually meant an all-day meeting, and often a meeting in a grove, and it drew white and black alike, sometimes almost in equal numbers. Another demand in this case—for the slaves knew how to make their demands—was that the negro preacher "should preach the funeral" as they called it. In things like this, the wishes of the slaves usually prevailed. "The funeral" loomed up weeks in advance, and although marked by sable garments, mournful manners and sorrowful outcries it had about it hints of an elaborate social function with festive accompaniments.
>
> *(Ibid., pp. 201–202)*

Recognizing the continued tradition of funeral rites as part of an African related rite of passage is important to seeing the underlying philosophical basis of an African diaspora life. In the discussion of slaves, former African American ancestors and rites of passage, there is an invocation of that which belongs to the spiritual realm.

A depth psychological perspective assumes that there can be an ancestral lineage through our archetypal DNA. Who can say whether this energy or pattern is only of a goddess or belongs to an ancestor, perhaps a combination of both? The significant matter is to accept that life does not begin and end with *one* life in one particular moment—except on a physical plane. In applying this idea to that of the rites of passage of life and death, we see cultural patterns that were crucial in keeping African Americans together as a unit and family, even when not related by blood, while slavery itself worked in the most careless fashion to rip apart this connection. The drawing of connections between African customs and African American rituals related to death and life establish more clearly and strongly a history that cannot be destroyed but lives in the archetypal lineage of the Middle Passage survivors.

In her discussion of funeral customs in *African American Funeral and Mourning Customs in South Carolina*, Elaine Nichols notes the following:

> The Bakongo people of Angola and the Congo were one of the groups that were enslaved and carried to South Carolina in significant numbers and whose burial customs are revealed in the past and present behaviors of African Americans. According to Robert Ferris Thompson the Bakongo believed that inanimate objects and things in nature had a living, conscious force within them, and that it was important to satisfy the spirit of the deceased and protect the living from the actions of dissatisfied spirits. The grave was a charm or powerful talisman that controlled events in the spirit world (world of the dead), as well as the world of the living. Objects placed on graves and rituals performed at the grave activated the grave's power. Objects were placed on burial sites to prevent spirits from wandering in search of any articles in the world of the living.
>
> *(2015, pp. 2–3)*

The significance of the aliveness of the energy of the grave is, I believe, directly related to the inter-connection between living and dead, archetypal and ego.

As the African American diaspora embraces it cultural heritage, always working to reshape meaning and significance, there is a need to include the spiritual and non-materialistic element of Africanist patterns. These would include references to passages of death and life since both were so heavily influenced in an unpredictable way by American slavery. In the same way in which slavery impacted the physical bodies of the African diaspora, so too could slavery have had an influence on the archetypal. This influence moved through not only the earth-bound recognition of death but also the archetypal energy of a living energy which does not die. The emotions of an archetypal grief passes through not only the physical body of the remaining survivors but also the ethereal lives of the ancestors, their grave objects and whatever remains of a previous life. This interconnection permits and encourages a fluidity of energy that really is archetypal.

In closing this section, I cite once again from Nichols:

In western and central Africa the circle is an important religious and cultural element, especially in mortuary traditions that honor the dead. The circle is incorporated into art as well as dance. Known as circle dances in Africa and in South Carolina and other African American communities, the counterclockwise movement combined music with dancing/shouting and was identified as "plantation walk-arounds," "shouts," and "ring shouts." In the United States they were initially performed around graves and later in churches and at religious ceremonies. Jonathan C. David notes that they were most often performed in religious services "after a formal prayer meeting or preaching service."

Although the high point of African American ring shouts was probably during the late nineteenth century, they continued to survive through the twenty-first century.

(2015, p. 3)

I believe that the interweaving of cultural patterns of rites of passage in Africa and America address the archetypal significance of intergenerational psychic characteristics that include ideas and customs as well as emotions. Everything of culture from the African diaspora that may have been disregarded due to slavery and its aftermath belongs in a sacred space of regard in this our contemporary life. This includes ownership of rites of passage that include the emotional inheritance of grief surrounding intergenerational cultural trauma and loss.

4

SLAVERY AS ARCHETYPE AND THE PRAYER OF FREEDOM

The nature of slavery

Slavery has existed for thousands of years and did not begin with the institution of American slavery. The simplicity of this fact belies and I believe detracts from the painful experiences of those caught in the African Holocaust. There are those in our times who state this fact without any acknowledgement of the trauma of slavery to those enslaved for centuries and their descendants. As I write these words, many of us living in today's world see more clearly than ever the results of slavery on our racial, political and economic status. It seems that slavery and its history in relation to people of color has been sufficiently distorted and negatively portrayed to the extent that we have been separated from the realities of considering slavery itself. This lack of willingness to see and examine slavery, especially American slavery, has kept us safe in a way. It has kept it out of our consciousness and removed us from any experience of guilt, retribution or grief. Certainly, in America we have been able to hide behind a drive to *move forward* away from the history of slavery and its traumatic effects. This can and has worked in some instances for decades—especially for those whose ancestors were not brought over on slave ships or who were among the first generations to work on American slave plantations.

My words are not written here in an accusatory way but in a way that simply acknowledges the facts of how we have hidden in an American collective from the history of slavery and its American aftermath. In a previous book I have addressed American racial complexes, and the collective racial amnesia that plagues us to forget the emotional pain of our history of American slavery (Brewster, 2017, pp. 24–30).

It would be impossible to enter a discussion regarding the the traumatic grief and the highly emotional state of women of color without considering slavery itself, and the environment that has raised emotions to the level of archetypal grief.

In thinking about slavery, we understand first that it is a relationship of master to slave. It is a composition of human to human relations in which one person has power, control and in the case of American slavery, the acceptance of this societal circumstance with the approval of *all* societal institutions. This circumstance is oppressive to the very psychology of the group of individuals who are enslaved. The added element to American slavery was that hope was lost very close to the first generation of the arrival of slaves to America. Unlike in other parts of the world and in earlier times of slavery where there was hope of eventually freeing oneself and/or one's family from slavery, America's economic growth became exceedingly dependent on the bodies of African American slaves working on slave plantations. Though in the period prior to the Emancipation Proclamation and the Civil War some slaves were granted their freedom, millions remained enslaved for generations.

It could appear that the longevity of slavery without hope of release in your lifetime or your child's lifetime or that of your grandchildren, could cause the development of a condition such as being bound by archetypal grief.

Can you imagine the weight of the knowledge that your life was bound to rising at 5 a.m., eating scraps or little better, going to the fields to pick cotton, tobacco or take care of rice fields; working all day until sundown with men with whips whose job it was to beat you and keep you in the fields; returning to a shack where you fell onto a straw bed for your night's rest. Then to begin this life all over again the next day unless you were sold to another plantation and your day now included only the interruption of walking miles to the new plantation—leaving mother, husband or children behind.

I ask you to imagine this because this story of American slavery is one which we are not taught in most of our history books. The sorrow of the African American slave has gone untold for centuries because I believe the greatness of the sorrow was too overwhelming to bear. This was not the only reason—the shame of how this abuse had been perpetrated on millions also had to be denied. The racism of slavery moved underground and continues to survive in our institutions. This is reflective of what we are facing today in our society—the political eruptions of Charlottesville, the rise of the white supremacy movement and the continued death of African Americans within the context of violence perpetrated by police officers.

Our failure to be willing to recognize the effects of slavery on millions of people of color through apology or reparations continuously forces us to revisit the ghosts and shadows of American slavery.

I do believe that we are now beginning to have a barely whispered voice which is telling us as a society that we cannot move forward on a way which leads to forgetfulness of the history of American slavery. A very significant aspect of this inability to change our collective language and behavior as regards our racial lives in America is because slavery is archetypal and all the accompanying events following the invention of American slavery are tied to the psychic as well as the emotional and spiritual lives of all Americans. When we consider slavery as a continuous event that has happened over hundreds of years with the dynamic of one individual or groups that are subservient to another, in any combination of ethnic mix, we could be viewing this event within the context of Jung's words:

> The archetypes are not whimsical inventions, but autonomous elements of the unconscious psyche which were there before any invention was thought of. They represent the unalterable structure of a psychic world whose "reality" is attested by the determining effects it has upon the conscious mind.
> (CW9i, para. 451)

American slavery and its negative attributes continue to live in our collective unconscious, personal conscious and cultural being. As mentioned above, our unwillingness to face the history of slavery—our collective denial—presents major issues for resolving the emotional impact of slavery on our society. A second but equally important aspect of slavery is the physical elements of slavery practices. That human beings were held as a commodity for economic gain has greatly undermined the relationship between African American families and the American economic system.

The devaluation of Africanist people began even before they had left Africa. The dehumanizing fact of slavery presented a psychological insistence on the decreased value *of* the African body while promoting a monetary value *for* the slaveholder.

This type of hypocrisy was engaged in over centuries as human beings were sold, enslaved and held in torturous bondage. The hypocrisy of the above also showed itself in terms of American religious institutions. The fact of making Africanist people "savages" and "primitives" requiring salvation from their own heathen religious experiences was one of the most hypocritical instances of the institution of slavery. It has been noted that this particular aspect of American slavery was a major influence in justifying the continuation of slavery long past the point when foreign empires such as Britain and France had discontinued and outlawed slavery. The American colonies adhered to the continuation of slavery because of its profitability and their reliance on an Africanist population that could be portrayed as fit only for slavery because its people were "soulless."

Other aspects that show the nature of American slavery included the violation of human kindness through the destruction of Africanist families. From the very early days of slavery, family members were separated from one another through death or being sold off to different slave owners and plantations. Over time it became more of an accepted practice to keep children as long as possible with some extended or known distant relative family member for the early upbringing of the African American child. However, these relationships were always at the discretion of the slave owner. Neither mother nor child were ever guaranteed that they would remain together for their entire lives.

In fact, it was generally accepted that they would probably not spend their lives together. I believe that this aspect of the nature of American slavery created a pathway for a kind of grief that developed over centuries, and was particular to the existence and promotion of slavery. I believe that within human consciousness, which Knox speaks of as the possibility of an image schema for "containment" as opposed to an innate mother archetype, we can have outside of a consistent ego awareness—an aspect of the unconscious that recognizes oppression and shows itself in our behavior. When intensified at a collective level it presents as slavery or human bondage. In those who are enslaved the emotional impact would be exceptionally strong. How can we begin to imagine this emotional impact except in terms of an archetypal potentiality?

Archetypal complexity and simplicity

It might seem simplistic to express an idea regarding slavery as an archetypal event in the human unconscious. When thinking about Jung's theory of the archetypes I found it necessary to find my own way through considerations of his concepts and those post-Jungians who have followed him. I'm eager to know more and to find avenues and paths within Jung's theories that can be even more helpful to me and to the patients with whom I work. It is partly due to Jung's initial work on the unconscious that I am able to engage in and enjoy the clinical and exploratory work in which I am able to participate.

As a Jungian analyst, I prefer to see human, ego and unconscious patterns as related to a psychosocial paradigm. This fits within my own cultural complex and that of my ancestral family. I also believe that cognition and epigenetics can play a role in the intergenerational transmission of family group traits. I am not bound to either way of conceiving of how information moves from one generation to another and I also know that all that can be seen is not relayed through the biological sight of only my physical eyes. My ability to remain conscientious of how I choose to honor ancestors, see the limits of any Eurocentric-based psychology and engage in spiritual practices that create a personal psychological balance center are highly important.

How complex or simple is the idea of the archetypes? Jung felt that he had proven one certain aspect of the collective that was not racial but rather universal. As our knowledge regarding culture deepens, we can see how this would be a correct position. Jung believed that the archetype took its "clothes" from the culture in which it showed itself. This coloring of the archetype was a direct reflection of the culture consciousness at the archetype at the time of visibility to ego consciousness. The only difficulty was that early American Jungian psychology's inclusion of the *nigredo* (the color black) had as its application only negative sociological implications for Africanist people (Brewster, 2017).

The color of depth psychology

As we think about skin color, how do we as depth psychologists position ourselves? Do we have a particular privilege in being depth psychologists? Depth psychology gives us a certain kind of freedom—our belief in psyche and the unconscious gives us freedom. Thich Nhat Han wrote a very small, slim book that developed from his work with prisoners. He believed that through meditation one could free the mind. As depth psychologists, I think that we are fortunate to know the power of the imagination. We can imagine freedom but I sometimes wonder how we can bring others along with us. How does Individuation allow for the joining with others so that everyone is free? No one is truly free until everyone achieves freedom. How do we consider making this happen as depth psychologists? How do we perceive freedom as American depth psychologists? If we look at the history of depth psychology we can understand its European roots without too much difficulty. The lens through which we have been experiencing it since its infusion into American society has been clear and white.

Unlike other psychologies, depth psychology has found it difficult to add those of color to its lens except as Other. Its ability to see the possible inclusion that made up America's multicultural society has been missing, almost invisible. This is one of the features of keeping power and control, especially when as Jung says, there can be a fear of "going black." However, as post-Jungians we must find a way to relinquish fear of the dark and go into the *nigredo*. This first entry is the Self. Here we can begin to see the ways in which we have split ourselves into two parts and also see the coloring of ourselves which must change.

This inner seeing is shadowed by racial complexes. Jung says we can never get rid of our complexes; I imagine that we can only befriend them in a way that keeps us sane.

As we learn more about our racial complexes, as we teach ourselves how to see racially in a different manner, we begin to understand how those who joined mass movements must have transformed themselves. I imagine that freedom requires an internal transformation of psyche. This internal change would, I imagine, cause one to see color differently—skin color. It would mean accepting that color does matter, while not mattering for the cause for which you are struggling—your respected humanity, because it is your birthright. Everyone who joins the movement brings his/her differences which supports the creation of a bonding group held together by an authentic purpose—to imagine freedom.

The work of depth psychology and those in the field must be to begin with a vision of what they want depth psychology to become. The lens of whiteness can no longer hold. It is exclusionary. It is unconscious to see whiteness and only whiteness. A mass movement requires all colors. But Jung seemed to have a mistrust of the masses. He wrote often enough about modern man and the difficulty he (mostly he—not she) faced with a loss of religious foundations of the church and loss of his soul.

Jung's primary experience of the masses was of course during two exceptional experiences of world wars. The vividness with which he explored his premonition dreams of the First World War fills his autobiographical material. But as Jungians have we followed too closely in our fear of the masses?

Any leader who believes in freedom and a psychology of liberation says that we require masses—thousands, perhaps millions—who will join and participate in the necessary actions for freedom. How does this equate with Jung's view of the need for Individuation above that for joining with the masses or the group? Participation Mystique warns of an unconsciousness, a lowering of good ego function that could become an obsession if one is not careful—if one is seduced by the "primitive." In balancing our perspective on Jung, in fairness, we must allow that Jung also believed that Individuation requires and has its own demand for a return to the collective. One is not allowed the luxury of sitting in quiet contentment, enjoying our individuated state but must give something back to others—our work is to increase consciousness. I take this to mean that I have an obligation to do whatever I can, wherever I find shadow that harms another, to step forward. I am not offering myself as a martyr though many, many others have died fighting for freedom. Rather, I am advocating for what I believe Jung intended when he spoke of the one who returns—the hero returning to the village with something of value for sharing. I know it is arguable that this model of the hero returning adds to the Eurocentric model of hero being heroic and giving to the oppressed from high above. But I would argue that the hero or heroine exists in all cultures. And I do believe that there is such a thing as a calling. It is in the personalizing of my work based on my ethnicity, my cultural heritage and my sociopolitical "life" that guide my work.

The color of depth psychology then becomes infused with multiple possibilities for learning how to not just tolerate the masses—not just as a visitor but as one who truly lives with the grit of poverty, lack of education and roughness that masses offer in a possible change of consciousness. In the section on "One of the Lowly" in the *Red Book*, Jung relates a vision-story about a man he meets in an inn:

> After dinner I go to bed in a humble room. I hear how the other settles into his lodging for the night next door. He coughs several times. Then he falls still. Suddenly I awaken again at an uncanny moan and gurgle mixed with a half-stifled cough. I listen tensely—no doubt, it's him. It sounds like something dangerous. I jump up and throw something on. I open the door of his room. Moonlight floods it. The man lies still dressed on a sack of straw. A dark stream of blood is flowing from his mouth and forming a puddle on the floor. He moans half choking and coughs out blood. He wants to get up but sinks back again—I hurry to support him but I see that the hand of death lies on him. He is sullied with blood twice over. My hands are covered with it. A rattling sigh escapes from him. Then every stiffness loosens, a gentle shudder passes over his limbs. And then everything is deathly still.
>
> *(2009, p. 266)*

Once again in service to Jung I would like to reproduce a few more words from the same section:

> At your low point you are no longer distinct from your fellow beings. You are not ashamed and do not regret it, since insofar as you live the life of your

fellow beings and descend to their lowliness/you also climb into the holy stream of common life, where you are no longer an individual on a high mountain, but a fish among fish, a frog among frogs.

(Ibid., p. 237)

Though the image is of fish, we understand that Jung has a positive relatedness towards fish from his previous religious references to fish and Christianity. It is no blasphemous thing to have humanity swim together en masse. This simple example from Jung seems refreshing in considering that he is at times oppositional in his own thinking and descriptive language, causing us to wonder what he really believes regarding any particular situation.

In the field of depth psychology, we are followers of Jung—post-Jungians. As we move through the oftentimes muddy waters of racial references we may encounter in Jung's theories, we are not necessarily trying to keep Jungian psychology as it has been—that would be a great difficulty for us in today's world—but we must find ways of pushing against the history not just of Jungian psychology, but of American psychology in general.

This is what I consider the most important work to be done today. I think it is why we are here today. We are trying to think, feel, imagine ways into a wider deepening of the color of depth psychology. The challenge of continuing to move on while holding onto the past is an arduous one. I have within me the DNA of ancestors who were not only slaves but slaves who built a hugely successful plantation system that made many white families wealthy.

My bloodline carries the strength of all those before me who survived the auction blocks, the rice plantations and the whip of the overseer. When I can hold it, mine is the long perspective on history. Four hundred years is a very, very long time.

I am one of four African American Jungian analysts who have faced racial discrimination within the Jungian community. This is not a fantasy. It is an aspect of life being a person of color in any American institution. Probably since its inception, there has been a willingness for color blindness to keep Jungian psychology safely cocooned away from the harsh realities of the egoic collective wake state—poor American racial relations. Dreams and the archetypal can be very seductive. We understand this. It might have been easier to follow Jung's lead and walk away from the complications of American psychology. I say these things from an insider's perspective.

This perspective offers something of the voice of Other, within the context of cultural consciousness and differences in culture. Deepening within our psychology depends on finding a way to hold the strength of the history that is Jung's legacy while searching through other ways that tell the stories of those who bring color to depth psychology. This color not only represents skin culture but what this culture actually means from the lived racial experiences of ancestors and today's African diaspora.

The voice of the ancestors

Freedom requires a recognition of all that has preceded it or it is meaningless. In the African American psyche, slavery and freedom as archetypal events both preceded the African Holocaust. Freedom is a journey on a rocky road with travelers who are still present in spirit. The continuous struggle of the African diaspora for freedom once leaving Africa acknowledges the history of a journey that has not ended. Ancestors add their voices to the journey. These voices are the ones who first came to America in coffles—former slaves.

Pray for freedom: Abolitionism

The history of the Abolitionist movement began on the European continent in 1315 when the then king of France, Louis X, abolished slavery. The king of Spain, Charles 1, also declared an end to slavery to take place in 1542; however, this law was never passed in all the colonial states. Creating laws for colonies at such a huge distance from Europe almost assured that compliance would be an issue—long before the American Revolutionary War.

The official beginning of the Abolitionist movement that was to have the most influential effect on Africanist, colonized people occurred when in England at the end of the 18th century British and then American Quakers became interested and involved in the question of morality as related to the reality of slavery. In 1772, a legal case entitled the Somersett case, involved setting a fugitive slave free based on English common law which stated that slavery was forbidden and therefore no one could be held in slavery. This case set the precedent for English men such as Granville Sharpe and William Willberforce.

Slavery was officially abolished in all the American northern states in 1804. International slave trade was abolished in 1807 by America and Great Britain; the British Slavery Abolition Act of 1833 abolished slavery throughout the British Empire.

This is the legal background of initial European attempts to end the slavery of Africanist people. The underpinning of this movement was the Enlightenment with its focus on natural law—the idea that human beings did not require divine intervention in order to make the best decisions for themselves with regard to injustice, social life and freedom. Nature could be understood without the assistance of God. Slavery had been justified by the proposition that God wanted and desired some people to be enslaved; this idea came under question as the movement for the abolition of slavery became stronger in the years before the American Revolution. With the outbreak of the American Revolution, based politically and philosophically on the tenets of the Enlightenment, the idea of slavery as outdated and harmful to the American political psyche was taken up by Thomas Jefferson. We are getting the irony here, right? Natural law under the Enlightenment also believed in the protection of private property. Jefferson never gave up his slaves.

The religious fervor of what became known as the Great Awakening had a major influence on the growth and survival of the Abolitionist movement.

In *Holy Warriors: The Abolitionists and American Slavery*, James Brewer Stewart says the following:

> Among slaves and free blacks, the Great Awakening called forth powerful lay preachers whose messages of hope sustained the slave community and whose powerful oratory established enduring modes of expression for African American activists. By placing the voice of conscience over law, free will over original sin, and mutual benevolence over divine retribution, many Protestants, white no less than black, began groping toward a new vision of spiritual and personal liberty.
>
> *(1997, p. 14)*

The first American Abolitionists who gave strength to the movement came from a religious base of Christians who believed that slavery was "a moral abomination." These Quakers gained even greater strength for their intense focus on slavery and the need for America to rid herself of it as American patriots moved further away from England and closer to freeing themselves from British rule.

As war with England became more evident so did the discrepancy between white American patriots seeking freedom while holding African Americans in slavery. This contradiction became a fire that began to burn even brighter as 1776 drew closer. The contradiction continued into 1787 when the Constitution became a reality. When America's Founding Fathers began to draw up a constitution it became important to them that Southern plantation owners—land owners—should continue to have political and social power. This resulted in what had at first appeared to be a concern for liberty and equality for all men becoming a document that assured this only for white male property owners. Slaves would not be afforded the protection of a federal constitution because they were not property owners and were in fact themselves the property of white men.

Following the American revolution, and into the early years of the 1800s, the Abolitionists became more powerful. In December 1833, a small group of them met in Philadelphia and formed the American Anti-Slavery Society. This organization was committed to the immediate liberation of all American slaves. During the years that followed, they were known as the *immediatists*. The men that were founders of this group included William Lloyd Garrison, Lewis Tappan, James Birney and Elizur Wright. They were to be the leaders of the Abolitionist movement for the next thirty years.

Owing to their efforts anti-slavery societies were formed across the country. Oberlin College in Ohio was the first interracial American college which could be attended by blacks and whites, men and women, could attend. As the publisher of the *Liberator* newspaper Garrison rose to be the leading supporter of other publications which spoke powerfully against slavery. Due to the combined efforts of newspapers, public speeches and the involvement of church preachers, the movement gained many supporters from different classes of people—New York bankers to western New York farmers. A major reason for this was still the underlying message of religion in the form of "moral suasion." The argument was for the immediate release of all slaves from bondage based on the moral fact that slaves were entitled to their freedom.

Many more Americans began to listen to the Abolitionist message but there was fear and anxiety regarding the way in which slaves would be released. During the 1840s, slave ship mutinies became more common. The *Amistad* was wrecked on the shore of Long Island after slaves rebelled and killed her crew. A legal fight took place over the question of what to do with these black men. They were eventually defended in the Supreme Court by John Quincy Adams, and once freed, the men were sent back to Africa.

This ship rebellion and others that followed preceded the anti-slavery rebellions that took place under men such as John Brown and Denmark Vesey. Such local armed protests against slavery struck fear into the hearts of Southern planters equally as well as Northern whites who had arrived in America with their own biases against blacks.

As 1860 drew closer the Abolitionists were deeply involved in politics in support of their own candidate from the anti-slavery Liberty Party. Abraham Lincoln won the election even though as history has taught us his intention was not to free the slaves but rather to hold the American union together. According to Stewart, once the Civil War began the work of the Abolitionists became to create agreement between what had been two opposing forces—Southern and Northern. This was actually the beginning of the end of the immense power that the movement had held for over twenty-five years. When the Civil War ended, men from the movement joined the federal government in providing much-needed support for African Americans in gaining the rewards of their freedom. The establishment of the Freeman's Bureau was a result of Abolitionist intervention.

Lewis Bonner, a former slave offers us a view into that time after the Civil War:

> When the War was over, Master told us, "You are free now, jest like I am, and as you have no places to go, you can stay on and work on halvers." We stayed on three years, after slavery. We got little money, but we got room and board and didn't have to work too hard. It was 'nuf difference to tell you was no slaves anymore.
>
> (Cited in Mellon, 1988, p. 353)

The nature of freedom

Freedom is also an archetype. For generations—centuries—it has been given history, measure, weight and archetypal energy through the embodiment of women and men for generations, for centuries. The occurrence of slavery appeared to deny that freedom to certain people—especially Africanist. The intergenerational nature of American slavery tended to make freedom invisible. Slavery was abolished for only a select few. Then freedom began to emerge from the Africanist cultural collective.

When Jung spoke of the opposites that reside in human consciousness, noting how they can pull us apart within ourselves as well in our othering with those who are different from us, it seemed important to consider what becomes the opposite of slavery. Without an archetype of freedom, the African diaspora would still be enslaved—held in physical bondage. I think it is important to present this concept as the opposite of slavery because I believe it can be influential in creating a conscious, intentional movement that represents an idea that always existed in the minds of early Africans who were transported to America. It existed too in the consciousness of African Americans as they lived within the bounds of slavery.

Since their arrival in America in around 1619, African people had legally resisted slavery. Thus, from the beginning they were "stamped," or categorized, as criminals. In all of the fifty suspected or actual slave revolts reported in newspapers during the American colonial era, resisting Africans were nearly always cast as violent criminals, not people reacting to enslavers' regular brutality, or pressing for the most basic human desire: freedom (Kendi, 2016, p. 69).One of the falsehoods of slavery was that African Americans were docile and had no purposeful idea regarding freeing themselves from slavery. I believe this false idea was one of many which were used not only in service of keeping Africanist people from thinking about freedom but also to continue a negative consistent commentary about the personality of black people. This has been the ongoing narrative of the African diaspora.

There was no way in which those invested in slavery and post-Civil War racist practices were going to allow black people to have any dignity. An aspect of decreasing dignity and humiliating them was the creation of falsehoods pertaining to their characters and personalities. In addition to their being treated as criminals, Africanist people were also labeled as lazy. The caricature of this personality defect was captured by "Sambo." This stereotype child/man was the image of the black masculine that suited a white American fantasy. David Brion Davis in reiterating historian Stanley Elkins' definition of "Sambo" says the following:

> Sambo, the typical plantation slave, was docile but irresponsible, loyal but lazy, humble but chronically given to lying and stealing; his behavior was full of infantile silliness and his talk inflated with childish exaggeration. His relationship with his master was one of utter dependence and childlike attachment: it was indeed this childlike quality that was the very key to his being.
>
> *(2006, p. 51)*

A counter-argument presented by Davis is the response to Elkins given by historical sociologist Orlando Patterson:

> The Sambo ideology …. is not more realistic a description of how slaves actually thought and behaved than was the inflated conceptions of honor and sense of freedom an accurate description of their masters. What was real was the sense of honor held by the master, its denial to the slave, its enhancement

through the degradation of the slave, and possibly the slave's own feeling of being dishonored and degraded.

(Ibid., p. 52)

It has been argued successfully and also not successfully that the behavior of African men and women trapped in centuries-long slavery was shaped by the slavery experience itself. There was no psychological reward derived from providing excellent labor to white slave owners.

I would imagine that survival and freedom were the most important concepts that shaped Africanist thinking for all the time that they were enslaved. If we think that pain or pleasure is the way in which we are most driven as human beings then certainly Africanist people experienced the former in a decisive manner.

This being so, the intention of the slave's life would have been to escape into salvation—freedom—in this case the very absence of the pain of slavery. The behavior of enslaved African Americans would have followed their logical thinking—there was no reward for excelling at their labor on a slave plantation. For them, the most important reward would have been freedom either in the form of running away or death. A lesser possibility was to "slow down" the work and to be less productive. It has been noted that this became an aspect of survival until a better realized freedom of the body was likely. The "Sambo" child/man that the plantation owner desired to see was also very likely the Africanist slave, keeping some of their life energy for their own families. Everything would not and I suspect did not, go the slave owner. This can be seen by those African Americans and their descendants who managed to survive the plantations with some family members and skills to sustain them through the Reconstruction period. Their ability to preserve something of themselves through the following generations allowed the African diaspora to survive.

Freedom as an archetype itself creates a tension against the pull of slavery. The psychic energy that motivates some to want to enslave others does not exist in an archetypal vacuum. There will be created an equally energetic force in consciousness that wants to remedy, to balance the weight of slavery. I believe that freedom is what has emerged, given that it was already present in human consciousness as soon as slavery became apparent.

> As the sun fired up the sky on April 7, 1712, about thirty enslaved Africans and two Native Americans set fire to a New York building, ambushing the "Christians" who came to put it out, as the story was told. Nine "Christians" were slayed, five or six seriously wounded. The freedom fighters ran off into the nearby woods .... Fear and revenge smoldered through the city .... No matter what African people did, they were barbaric beasts or brutalized like beasts. If they did not clamor for freedom, then their obedience showed they were naturally beasts of burden. If they nonviolently resisted enslavement, they were brutalized.

If they killed for their freedom, they were barbaric murderers .... Their "barbarism" occasioned a "severe" slave code, resembling the laws passed by the Virginians and Puritans in 1705. New York lawmakers stripped free Blacks of the right to own property, and then they denigrated "the free negroes of the colony" as an "idle, slothful people" who weighed on the "public charge."

(Kendi, 2016, p. 70)

5

MOTHERING SLAVE AND THE INTERGENERATIONAL ORPHAN

Mothering slaves

The term *mothering slave* was created to define those African diaspora women who had been captured and put into slavery and used as reproduction females for the economic success and survival of the plantation system. The term designates these women because their purpose was for the birthing of Africanist children. The term first came to my attention at a conference held in 2016 entitled "Mothering Slaves: Maternity, Childlessness and the Care of Children During and After Slavery," and sponsored by the British Royal Historical Society. The conference was the first of its kind and sought to address the under-researched topic of enslaved women and their children.

Through the act of procreation women still fulfill a most important action for the survival of our human race. The intersection of race and sex produced a unique experience for the Africanist woman when she became the lynchpin for fueling economic success for centuries for whites in a racially exploitive system without benefiting from this system's success. She became the mother who could produce great success through the physical and psychological pain of being female and yet reap none of the rewards. She was unable to reap any of the monetary rewards of having been used as a "breeder" nor the psychological joy of having been a mother in the true sense of the word because her biological children were not her own—they were the property of others.

The cultural trauma of being at the center of slavery, as a mothering slave, was impactful from its onset. In the world of the slave mother, there was little room for compassion, because there was no room for weakness. This was especially true when the mother herself had been compromised. A Northerner who settled in Mississippi spoke with mothers who were concubines there: "They had too much pride and self-respect to rear their daughters for such a purpose," he said.

"If driven to desperation, she destroyed herself to prevent it, or killed them" (Giddings, 1988, p. 45).

Little has been written about this cultural trauma to the women who endured sexual assault and child production—as "breeders." We have only now begun to have conversations about cultural trauma to the broad collective of Africanist people—men, women and children who survived the Middle Passage and the plantations of slavery.

It is taking time to open our eyes and have a willingness to see into some experiences of American slavery. The women who lived on plantations and birthed our ancestors were indeed strong, resourceful and powerfully capable at ensuring a maternal line of survival. These are the women who produced children who helped us to gain freedom from slavery, enter the Industrial Revolution of the early 20th century and led us to the Civil Rights and Black Power movements that gave us judicial power. It was their focus on having their descendants understand the power of education that has brought African Americans middle- and upper-class status out of the painful poverty of slavery.

The continued invisibility of historical narratives about mothering slaves and the narrating of their stories speaks to the overall pattern of carelessness with which Africanist women were treated from the beginning of slavery when they were first brought to the Americas by the Portuguese.

It appears that there was never a time when the women of Africa were collectively treated without physical or mental abuse since their arrival in America. This includes the decades that followed the Civil War. The racist element that caused their initial landing at American slave ports has actually barely changed over the centuries. Yes, slavery has ended in its cruelest form but the unconscious undercurrent that accepted slavery, I believe, continues to live on in the American psyche cultural complexes.

Yes, the number of Africanist women who are raped as a hate crime with the overt *support* of the American judicial system has decreased since slavery. However, when I speak about the discrimination that African American women continue to experience in terms of their overall presence in America I am not speaking about their improved economic status. I'm also reflecting on the collective impressions, language, level of disrespect and other negativity shown by whites to Africanist women of color. The level of contempt and shaming—in lieu of whippings and verbal denigration directed at black women—remains palpable in the American collective unconscious. Melissa V. Harris-Perry takes up this idea in *Sister Citizen: Shame, Stereotypes, and Black Women in America*:

> Although Jim Crow drew a bright line of legislated shame around the entire race, women were particular targets. Victorian sensibilities held that women were uniquely endowed with morality and ethics. Because they held authority in domestic matters, women were considered the tender sex whose delicacy required special dispensation in public spaces. The special treatment of fragile women as a signal of civility, and those who treated women rudely or roughly

in public were labeled barbarians. But this courtesy was extended only to white women. Black women, regardless of class, education, or status, were potential targets of public abuse, ridicule, and mistreatment in the Jim Crow South. The permissible mistreatment of black women was a vicious form of collective shaming.

(2011, pp. 112–113)

A large part of the aspect of shaming that was projected onto black women was based on the development of viewing them as animals of labor. This connection of the idea that there existed human women as a lower form of animal life was initially developed as another rationale for slavery and holding them in bondage.

One of the most pronounced experiences and historical facts of black women is the comparison of their physicality to animals though this has generally been an aspect of slavery—treating humans like "beasts" from the early recorded days of slavery.

This feature was exaggerated and has persisted from slavery to the present day in terms of defining African Americans. From Davis's discussion of European explorers, we are able to obtain an understanding of their perception and characterization of black people:

> As Europeans continued to discover more "primitive" peoples on the planet, countless observers echoed the sixteenth-century English voyagers who described sub-Saharan Africans as "beastly savage people," "wilde men." And "brutish blacke people." An early French explorer wrote that Australian aborigines, who unlike the West Africans were still hunter-gatherers, were "the most miscrable people in the world, and the human beings who approach closest to brute beasts." With respect to the links between bestiality and slavery, from the earliest Sumerian tablets and other records dating from the mid-third millennium B.C.E., captive slaves have been equated with domesticated animals in pricing, status, and the way they have been described …. It is thus of immense importance that slaves, regardless of origins or ethnicity, were seen to carry the marks of childlike and animalistic inferiority later ascribed to such inferior peoples as Australians an sub-Saharan Africans.
>
> *(2006, pp. 52–53)*

Inhuman bondage: the rise and fall of slavery in the New World

From the earliest history of the capture of individuals into slavery we can see references to them as "domesticated animals." It is important to note that any females who were enslaved were not *intentionally* used as "breeders" for bringing more children into the slavery system. This was a feature of the African Holocaust. It was understood that the line of enslaved individuals followed the maternal lineage. Being born into slavery meant slavery for the child even when the father was white. One of the features of American slavery was its reliance on this idea of slavery following a maternal lineage. This worked very well for slaver owners who were economically invested in increasing the number of black children being born on their plantations. The "domestication" of American slaves became an aspect of slavery in the 1830s as the "new slavery" took shape.

Under this "new slavery" slaves were considered "human" and potentially able to be "tamed." They were not to be physically abused—they were only to be whipped for "wrong-doing." Unfortunately, this still depended on the white overseer, slave owners and any white family member's opinion as to what had been done "wrong." As this social idea of more acceptable treatment of African Americans took shape it did not really positively affect them in any way. Black women continued to be sexually assaulted and to produce both physical labor and children for the plantation.

The idea of Africans, including men, as originating from and being undeveloped ape-men was blatant in American society. Robert V. Guthrie in *Even the Rat Was White: A Historical View of Psychology* (2004) discusses the treatment of Africans at the St. Louis World Fair in 1904, a where series of "tests" measuring intelligence and motor skills were administered by members of the World's Congress of Races to African people from Senegal and the Congo.

The test results were predictable in ascertaining that those tested (which included Native Americans), were of lower intelligence and overall abilities than whites. Guthrie relates a rather understated event resulting from the fair that might be considered only a footnote by some but directly points to the racial attitude of equating Africans to animals:

> A tragic ending occurred when one of the fair's participants, Ota Benga from the Belgian Congo, unwittingly found himself later displayed in a monkey cage at the Bronx Zoo (New York). After a public brouhaha, Ota Benga was released from the zoo. Realizing he could never return to his motherland, Ota Benga later committed suicide in Lynchburg, Virginia.
>
> *(2004, p. 48)*

A photograph of Ota Benga and four other African men taken at the time of the fair show him with a monkey standing in front of and holding onto him. None of the other men are standing with animals. Africans have historically been equated most often with the monkey and orangutan. This initially began in Africa and later traveled to the United States. Black women were not excluded from this animalistic characterization.

In *Ar'n't I a Woman: Female Slaves in the Plantation South*, Deborah Gray White elaborates this idea:

> How white Americans, and Southerners in particular, came to think of black women as sensual beings has to do with the impression formed during their initial contact with Africans, with the way black women were forced to live

under chattel slavery, and with the ideas that Southern white men had about women in general …. Even in the Chesapeake, ideas about promiscuous black women held firm. Suggesting that black women mated with orangutans, Thomas Jefferson was certain that this animal preferred "the black woman over those of his own species."

(1998, pp. 29–30)

This idea of Africanist female bestiality did not, however, prevent Thomas Jefferson from "mating" with Sarah Heming, African American slave half-sister to his wife. The hypocrisy of the American white collective was brilliantly on display during and after slavery.

The constructed view of Africanist women was developed by whites in service of creating two major stereotype versions of black women—the *jezebel* and the *mammy*. We are familiar with both of these mythological figures as they have appeared in American language and images for over a century. The white American collective psyche had to create a psychological fixture, an identifying container for the black women. History suggests that they knew little to nothing of the actual culture, attributes or African societies from which black women came and as previously noted the small amount they knew was distorted and largely misunderstood. The creation of a jezebel stereotype was not difficult based on the conscious promoted thinking of black women as hypersexualized beings. The rape of black women gained a societal rationale and acceptance because of black women's own sexual behaviors. Men were at a disadvantage when interacting with black women in terms of controlling their sexual urges. This idea worked to weave a story of racist intrigue and seduction that permitted black women to become the whorish opposite of virtuous white women—jezebels. They could then be limitlessly preyed upon as sexual objects.

The other image of black women that has dominated American collective consciousness for over a century is that of the mammy. As African Americans gained greater psychological freedom to truly access their own capacities following Reconstruction and as a result of the Black Power movement of the 1960s, an important realization (once again), was the significance of how selected racist symbols had grown in usage in America. Like the jezebel stereotype, the mammy one was built on a tiny detail relating to black women and was then expanded to suggest a role that was severely distorted.

In the jezebel stereotype, black women had been created as extremely oversexed individuals. Within this false message was an accompanying one that they deserved to be sexually assaulted because of their promiscuity. They were no more sexual than any other human being, black or white, but rather had been racially sexualized in the service of racial economics and other human failures. The detail about the jezebel symbol of black women that grew beyond any ethical standard and was psychologically abusive to African American women was that they were sexually insatiable and needed to have sexual relations with any man, as well as with animals. The despairing detail is that this became one of only two possibilities of which they were capable as women. The jezebel was well suited for sexual assault with procreation as an acceptable outcome. The other possibility was that of the mammy.

The minute detail of truth about the mammy was that once past the age to produce children for slave owners, she was delegated to being the housekeeper, cook, childcare substitute mother, sometime-field hand and any other role required by the white owners for whom she worked. According to Deborah Gray White:

> She was a woman completely dedicated to the white family, especially to the children of that family. She was the house servant who was given complete charge of domestic management. She served also as friend and advisor. She was, in short, surrogate mistress and mother.
>
> *(1998, p. 49)*

It became increasingly possible for aging black women to fill this role as they were restricted by slavery from being anything else. At each end of a human relation spectrum in slavery black women could either be a jezebel—a whore/child-producing woman, or a grandmother—mammy. In consideration of the archetype she was never the Virgin Mary, nor a goddess. She was always a woman who had been imaginatively overly sexualized as a young woman or the older black woman who was no longer useful for love (except by white children and their parents—whom she might also have raised), nor for sexual relations in order to procreate.

When we consider what sort of person or personality we might be drawn to, having a mammy would be one of our first choices. She was supposedly a woman full only of love and kindness for her white family. What of her black family? Her own children she had in many cases already lost to the slave auction, or had been given as a "gift" to a white family member, or had died due to the effects of slavery. This was a deeper shadow side of being a mammy. There are numerous pictures of black women mammies holding white babies. How did she hold her own children? When did she hold them? Where are the historical pictures of black women holding their own children?

> One of the key figures in the white child's socialization was the ubiquitous black mammy to whom he frequently turned for love and security. It was the black mammy who often ran the household, interceded with his parents to protect him, punished him for misbehavior, nursed him, rocked him to sleep, told him fascinating stories, and in general served as his second, more attentive, more loving mother.
>
> *(Blassingame, 1972, p. 266)*

There are enough accounts by witnesses to slavery and by those who lived after those times to share the truth about the life of a mammy. Ultimately, the black women who worked as servants in the "big house" were still slaves. They may have been able to obtain somewhat better food to share with those living in shacks on the plantation or they might be given castoffs to wear, but they lacked their freedom and were bound to the lives of a white family—a family that was not their own. The attachment that these women may have felt for their white families I imagine would have developed out of fear, sadness as well as a need to survive. In her role as mammy, a black woman knew a great deal about white and black relationships on the plantation. She was privy to information not known by other African Americans who worked only in the fields and who never entered her predominately white workplace.

I wonder about the sadness and grief of the real jezebel and the mammy—not the constructed caricatures of thousands, perhaps millions, of black women. As young black girls came of age without rituals for this rite of passage, what prepared them for a future of sexual assault and the possible eventual removal of her future children into the chains of slavery? How did her grief pass from one generation of young women to another, all of whom became future mothering slaves?

When I speak of the focus on the physicality of African American women from the beginning of slavery until the present day I think that we can still see this fixation—even if collectively we wish to be in denial. It became possible during the presidency of Barack Obama and First Lady Michelle Obama to see in a very significant new and yet historical way, the treatment of African American women. The possibility of this circumstance was exceptional due to President and Mrs. Obama being the first African Americans to occupy such a position in American history. They would have to endure a great deal based on their ethnicity. The First Lady would have to carry all of the historical projections of any highly visible black woman and much more. When referring to an article written by Maureen Dowd for the *New York Times* entitled "Should Michelle Cover Up", Melissa V. Harris-Perry brings us to that remembrance of the American collective thinking, conscious and unconscious, of Africanist women:

> The piece was written in response to Michelle's having worn a sleeveless purple dress to President Obama's first address to a joint session of Congress. Dowd's article rehearses some familiar American anxieties about black women bodies. *She expresses a sort of terror that Michelle is a symbol of overt sexuality that should be covered and shrouded so as not to distract men of power* .... Dowd echoes the white women of antebellum plantations who fretted about maintaining the virtue of their husbands and sons in the presence of scantily clad enslaved women, who were thought to be sexually insatiable.
>
> *(2011, p. 278; emphasis in the original)*

As First Lady Michelle Obama provided new images, language and possibilities to the American racial psyche. I believe that her presence in the White House with her own two daughters will forever change the potentiality of unconscious events in terms of ethnicity and cultural complexes. I have included this short section about the former First Lady because I believe the election of her husband, Barack

Obama, and their family to the White House showed a shift in the collective unconscious of the archetype.

I believe that their lives as President and First Lady reflect a change in consciousness that we are currently seeing with the societal pendulum swing to Donald Trump. The events of Trump's presidency are so enormous at a collective egoic level that I imagine the return to a certain normalcy, driven from a collective unconscious, will be even greater than the results of the election of President Obama.

The intergenerational orphan

An orphan is a child who has been deserted or given away by his or her birth mother and/or father. Such a child may have been left at birth or not until many years later following this birth. We might say that an orphan a child who has been abandoned or left in the care of others. When I look for models in the American social system for helping to create a structure and language to identify the slavery experience by Africanist people, in my case women, I have difficulty finding a frame. I believe this is partly due to the fact of historical attempts to hide the truth of the genocidal nature of the African Holocaust.

I also think that finding a frame is difficult because I must consider a structure that has never existed before in terms of culture. It is very similar to exploring the five stages of grief and dying when it is intergenerational—what can possibly serve as a model for 400 years of intergenerational slavery, torture, death and grief?

The children of American slavery fit into different categories, and though facing the same basic suffering of slavery, had varying experiences of slavery. One thread of their experiences that ran through each of the lives of enslaved children was the breaking up of family even in the very presence of mothers and fathers.

In the beginning:

> In Africa, slave-ship captains assembled a live cargo over a period of weeks as local traders came downriver, sometimes waiting for a nearby battle to end so that war captives would be available for purchase. The captives' heads were shaved before they were packed belowdecks, a precaution against lice that also de-individualized them, along with stripping them of their names, identities and culture. Likewise their clothes went: most were shipped naked, in violation of the traditional modesty of many African societies. The modern sense of a factory was already implicit in what the slave trade did. Through a series of dehumanizing procedures, it processed the raw material people into a value-added industrial product: slaves .... The systematic crushing of the black family by the later antebellum slave-breeding industry began with the severance of African family ties. The elite of the Americas, whose successive generations tended to remain elite, and who had in many cases come from Europe with the advantage of family connections, did everything possible to make sure that the family structures of Africa, which in some cases included royalty, high priests, and military heroes, did not transfer their webs to the Americas.
>
> *(Sublette and Sublette, 2016, p. 151)*

One very important element that keeps them together is the bond of the intergenerational cultural trauma of being without the stable, protected psychological presence of a home or family, even when a physical home/shack was provided by the slave owner. Slave children, even when living on the same plantation with their natural birth mothers, were most often without the "privilege" of truly being with them in any consistent kind of mother-child way. Their mothers may have wanted to protect them, feed them and love them as any mother would but these children learned that they could not have this type of relationship with their mothers without the interfering control of the slave owner. What is the psychological effect of such a situation? How do we measure despair not only for one child but for many over generations? I think this despair is the archetypal reflective grief of the child joining that of the mother, caught in a bond of sorrow. This bond is transformed over time with and by the conscious and unconscious grief of mothers and children caught by slavery.

Olaudah Equiano was an African stolen into slavery from his own front yard when he was a child. Both he and his sister were taken but were eventually separated. In 1789, Equiano wrote his memoir documenting his experiences upon being enslaved:

> The first object which saluted my eyes when I arrived on the coast was the sea, and a slave ship, which was then riding at anchor, and waiting for its cargo. These filled me with astonishment, which was soon converted into terror when I was carried on board. I was immediately handled and tossed up to see if I was sound by some of the crew, and I was not persuaded that I had gotten into a world of bad spirits, and that they were going to kill me.
> *([1791] 1995, p. 57)*

As the system of slavery developed, the children of this system could have different lives depending on how and when they arrived in America—brought as slaves in the early days or born later into slavery at the beginning of the emancipation. However, I believe that in this basic life as a slave was the archetypal event of being and becoming an orphan. A perpetual anxiety might exist in the life of a slave child, once she could understand that she belonged to someone—a slave owner or trader, while simultaneously belonging to no one—her birth mother. I believe that this hollow space created a sense of abandonment whether standing on an auction block or walking the plantation land of the father-slave owner. This is not the clearly defined *abandonment* of being left by birth parents so that they can have the freedom of their own lives without children.

Instead, it is the parental leave-taking, capturing and stealth of Africanist children into ownership by another. It is the rupture of families who wish to be together. These children are not abandoned in the way that we might think of abandonment and yet will have the loneliness and despair of having been left behind *as if* they were abandoned. They have been left but through no fault of their parents. They may have the experience of feeling abandoned and lost but it has not been done intentionally by their African parents.

Some children who had been stolen directly from Africa were able to remember and share their stories through oral narratives Following them were their descendants, grandchildren of Africans, who were born in America and could only listen to stories about the motherland. The children born of these stolen Africans were the first American generation slaves. Chaney Mack was one such African American:

> My father wuz a full-blooded African. He wuz about eighteen years old when dey brought him over. He come from near Liberia. He said his mother's name wuz Chaney, and dat's what I git my name. He said dat wasn't no winter whar he come from, and if dey felt like it dey could all go stark naked. He wore a slip made of skins of wild animals that come down to his knees. When ships would land in Africa, de black folks would go down to watch dem, and sometimes day would show dem beads and purty things dey carried on de ship. One day, when my daddy and his brother, Peter, wuz standing round looking, de boss-man axed dem if dey wanted to work and handed dem a package to carry on de boat. When dey got in dere, dey see so many curious things dey just wander aroun' looking, and before dey know it de boat has pulled off from de landing and dey is way out in de water and kain't he'p demselves. So dey jest brought 'em on over Georgy and sold 'em. Dem was a boat load of 'em, all stolen.
>
> *(Mellon, 1988, p. 49)*

Then came one generation after another born into slavery. The following are their voices:

> Ole Missus and young Missus told the little slave children that the stork brought the white babies to their mothers, but that the slave children were all hatched out from buzzards' eggs. And we believed it was true.
>
> *(Katie Sutton, former slave; ibid., p. 39)*

> De fus' thing I recollect is living in a a slave cabin back o' Marse's big house, along wid forty or fifty other slaves. All my childhood life, I can remember seeing my pa or ma gwine to wuk or coming in from wuk in de daylight, as dey went to de fiel's fo' day an' wukked till after dark. It was wuk, wuk, wuk, all de time. My ma wukked in de fiel's up to de day I was born. I wuz born 'twix de fiel's an' de cabins. Ma wuz den token to de house on a hoss.
>
> *(Jennie Webb, former slave; ibid., p. 35)*

> I was born in Georgia on a farm. My mother's name was Lucindy. I heard other Negroes say she was a good woman, but she died when I was a little boy, not more than three or four. She left my little brother a crawlin' baby 'bout eleven months old. I can remember a little her dyin'. I remember her

rockin' me on the steps and singin'. "Lord revive us. All our help must come from Thee." I can remember cryin' for my mama and bein' lonesome for her. They tried to tell me she was dead, but I couldn't get it through my little head.

(Jack Maddox, former slave; ibid., p. 115)

Finally, there were those children who were born into slavery and who were able to directly experience freedom from slavery after 1865. These emancipated African Americans were the first among the African diaspora in two centuries to know freedom due to the government intervention that set free all slaves.

I wuz pow'ful glad when I wuz freed. One thing they did wuz to whitewash de bullwhip and hang it on de side of de house.

(Hester Norton, former slave; ibid., p. 354)

The generational listing of these ancestors captures my attention, demanding that something be told of each one of their lives. These lives under slavery's yoke that began with the coffles in Africa. Even with the plantation system's pattern of keeping some families together, so many African American families were broken up and lost to one another forever. This is partially due to the long duration of American slavery and also to the fact of black people being thought of as dehumanized items for auction and sale—seeing Africans as having families was not a necessity for those capturing and selling them.

Each child born to an African mother, or, later, to an African American, risked being enslaved. Those who were not slaves at birth had been given away into freedom through the power and choice of a slave owner. The life and death of Africanist people was held by this man and many others like him. The stress of the possibility of death was always present in the psychological minds of slaves. Historical oral narratives show a line of anxiety that ran through most of these narratives.

All of the slaves in the narratives I explored for this book had witnessed violence towards other slaves or had themselves been the victims of violence. Oftentimes, they had seen this violence perpetrated against their own family members or individuals known to them. Frequently, this violence led to death. This was the life of the American slave. In the American collective, those of us of African ancestry are asked in various ways to let go of the past—to forget about this past that tore families apart, kept us impoverished for hundreds of years and that caused us to lose our children through the effects of slavery. First, we must know this past—the truth of it, before we can be expected to let go—if ever. Millions of people whose ancestors have experienced a holocaust should not be expected to relinquish their past, their cultural trauma. Never forgetting is for *all* holocaust victims—this certainly includes the African Holocaust.

The connections between mothering slaves and their children were tenuous and could be easily broken by anyone (white) outside their family, and for any capricious reason. The issue of a psychological abandonment experienced by these children could effectively pass through generations. The way in which African Americans were sold oftentimes left no way of knowing where one's family member had gone to—slaves had no right to this information. It was dependent upon the whim of the slave owner whether a slave could be allowed to know the whereabouts of family members. This became impossible if the person was being sent away—sold—due to the anger of the slave owner. The loss and ever-present threat of losing loved ones would have added an anxiety of separation that would remain in the Africanist psyche over generations.

This I identify as part of archetypal grief. It is the ever-present sorrow for those who have left without any foreknowledge of where they have gone or if they will be seen again. I believe that this level of consistent grief has the ability to change consciousness. It can influence the emotional state of each individual born into the next generation.

I find it both difficult and possible to imagine myself in the experience of my former ancestors. When I read their stories and remember the inflection of their Gullah voices, I see how I belong with them and they with me. When I dream about them or remember some personal habit, I know that I bring from these memories the archetypal potentiality of living and reliving a past that never dies but is passed on intergenerationally. These ancestral other lives reside in the unconscious. Allowing myself access to the truth that there is another truth that lives outside of my ego-wake state narrative supports a deepening within the unconscious spirit, and that which is not only visible to the physical eyes.

I believe that all of the children who were lost due to slavery continue to have the archetypal potential for sharing grief intergenerationally with Africanist women of color. This is slavery's legacy. Their grief does not just disappear into a black hole without recognition of meaning. Millions of children passed away without having experienced a normal emotional engagement with their mothers. How do we reconcile ourselves to this fact? Where do we carry sorrow like this in human consciousness? I believe that we must first acknowledge that such a thing existed. Our willingness to explore and accept this fact has been limited. This limitation and refusal to engage only deepens the frustration of wanting and needing to heal through remembrance.

Does each child of the African diaspora today carry, like a genetic factor, the possibility of inheriting at an archetypal level the racial potentiality—the racial complex, cultural complexes of which Jung initially spoke? Do the gods and goddesses speak to us within the dream, sharing what the ancestors might be desiring? Are we willing to see and hear at a more spiritual level the essence of the ancestor's voices?

The intergenerational orphan becomes every Africanist child because of the African Holocaust. Over the past century and a half we have failed to reach a state of equality in America which reflects racial peace and harmony at a collective level. This is a part of the reason why I say that each African American child remains an intergenerational orphan. When I address the issue of the psychological status of us as slave descendants this does not refer to more of the physical needs that have been better met since after the first years of slavery. Instead I'm speaking about the cultural pain inherited as the descendant of former slaves that continues to be unresolved. As stated earlier, I believe this remains unresolved because we as an American collective have been largely unwilling to permit remembrance of this cultural trauma. In the attempt at suppression, everything gets pushed back into the shadows and any activity to bring to light the darkness of racism that caused the cultural trauma is also critically forbidden or avoided. *This* is the American conversation I believe we are currently engaged in at a collective level. Until this shifts towards the direction of acknowledgement and awareness, our collective racial healing is delayed and each new generation is born into the repetitive cultural trauma of previous generations.

6

AFRICAN AMERICANS AND ELISABETH KÜBLER-ROSS

Stages of grief

An American awakening

When Elisabeth Kübler-Ross published her first book, *On Death and Dying*, Americans were surprised and awakened by the blunt honesty of her discussion of the topic of death and dying. In all of our American cultural awareness of death, I believe that we were still attempting to psychologically hide the fact of death away from our consciousness. In her introduction to the idea of our fear of death Kübler-Ross says the following:

> The ancient Hebrews regarded the body of a dead person as something unclean and not be touched. The early American Indians talked about the evil spirits and shot arrows in the air to drive the spirits away. Many other cultures have rituals to take care of the "bad" dead person, and they all originate in this feeling of anger which still exists in all of us, though we dislike admitting it. The tradition of the tombstone may originate in the wish to keep the bad spirits deep down in the ground .... Though we call the firing of guns at military funerals a last salute, it is the same symbolic ritual as the Indian used when he shot his spears and arrows into the skies. I give these examples to emphasize that man has not basically changed. Death is still a fearful, frightening happening, and the fear of death is a universal fear even if we think we have mastered it on many levels.
>
> *(1970, p. 5)*

Kübler-Ross's book brought more into our consciousness this aspect of an American shadow over our collective fear of death. In her Preface to the text, she says of her book:

> It is not meant to be a textbook on how to manage dying patients, nor is it intended as a complete study of the psychology of dying. It is simply an

account of a new and challenging opportunity to refocus on the patient a human being.

She continues:

> We have asked him (patient) to be our teacher so that we may find out about the final stages of life with all its anxieties, fears, and hopes.
>
> *(Ibid.)*

I find this to be a valuable attempt not only generally from a depth psychology perspective because Kübler-Ross has investigated these American emotions related to death, but also specifically for those of the African diaspora, who lived and died during slavery and its aftermath. I consider the benefits of a 20th-century theory regarding death and how we might use such a theory to bring comfort to the process of dying. I also think about ancestors and traditional African philosophy regarding death, and am drawn to conceptualize a different model for those of the African diaspora who left behind important rituals regarding the rite of passage of death in Africa. However, we have learned through careful study that not all African rituals and customs were lost. Many from this lineage have been discovered among the religious and funeral practices of African Americans. This has proven true even in my own personal family history. In the chapter on "Africanism in Secular Life," Herskovits discusses Puckett's research:

> What may be regarded as a generalized pattern of formal leave-taking of the dead by all his relatives and close friends, with varied rites during the process, is deeply rooted in West African funeral rituals. The custom of passing young children over the coffin has not been reported for West Africa, but something closely related to it has been witnessed among the Bush Negroes of Dutch Guiana .... In another case in South Carolina the children march around the father's casket singing a hymn, after which the youngest is passed first over and then under the casket and the casket is taken out on and run upon the shoulders of two men.
>
> *([1958] 1990, p. 205)*

I was eight years old when my paternal grandfather died. I remember that his body lay in a casket in the living (front) room of his home. A discussion took place between my parents and my grandmother concerning whether I should be passed over my grandfather's casket. The decision was made not to do this since it was felt that given my age, the fact that I had been baptized and was close enough to my grandfather in a loving relationship, it was unnecessary to pass me over his casket.

Herskovits says:

> The wake is as important in Africa as it is in the West Indies and the United States. It is reasonable, however, to suppose that as found in the New World it

is an example of the process of mutual reinforcement experienced when similar cultural impulses from two sources come into contact.

([1958] 1990, p. 205)

Ethnicity influences how we live and view dying. The African diaspora have certainly retained enough of their death and funeral rituals to have them marked and noted in America. My own personal experiences growing up in a small coastal town in South Carolina have allowed me to see the "mutual reinforcement" of Africanist traditions through the verbal and physical behaviors of my recent ancestors.

Though my parents and grandmother discussed the passing of my body over that of my recently deceased grandfather for my protection and continued life into adulthood, this ritual was for the ancestral peace of my grandfather as well as to bring peace in my own life.

John Mbiti in *African Religions and Philosophy* says:

> People know only too well that following physical death, a barrier has been erected between them and the living-dead …. The living-dead are wanted and yet not wanted. If they have been improperly buried or were offended before they died, it is feared by the relatives or the offenders that the living-dead would take revenge. This would be in the form of misfortune, especially illness, or disturbing frequent appearances of the living-dead.
>
> *(1989, p. 83)*

This family discussion took place in my presence and in the presence of my recently passed grandfather. My grandfather was still part of our family conversation and could contribute his "voice." His inclusion and mine were intentional.

Mbiti states:

> Because they are still "people", the living-dead are therefore the closest link between men and God: they know the needs of men, they have "recently" been here with men, and at the same time they have full access to the channels of communicating with God directly or, according to some societies, through their own forebearers. Therefore people may involve them in family affairs more often for minor needs of life than they approach God. Even if the living-dead may not do miracles or extraordinary things to remedy the need, men experience a sense of psychological relief when they pour out their hearts' troubles before their seniors who have a foot in both worlds.
>
> *(1989, p. 82)*

I believe that in my own father's sorrow and closeness to his father, he welcomingly sought his father's presence and saw no need to move the family discussion to a physical space that was separate from my grandfather.

Kübler-Ross: stages of death

In *On Death and Dying,* Kübler-Ross develops a theoretical concept regarding the stages of death that included emotional reactions to the death of another, especially a close family member or spouse. The five stages are denial, anger, bargaining, depression and acceptance. These stages were presented from the perspective of the terminal individual. Kübler-Ross followed up the publication of her first book, *On Death and Dying,* with several others on the same theme.

The last in her series regarding death, co-authored with David Kessler, is entitled *On Grief and Grieving: Finding the Meaning of Grief Through the Five Stages of Loss.* The authors state that they do not believe that all the stages might follow in a regulated, highly structured order. Each person grieves differently in accordance with their beliefs. Kübler-Ross and Kessler's model of grief does not take into account the cultural trauma of a particular group of people. The authors, who believe that there is no group experience to grieving, state that the five stages have been misinterpreted. This is one place of departure for me from the authors as I think about archetypal grief and cultural trauma. As we move within wider society it becomes clear that some people are more willing to accept the death and dying process and invite conversations about it into our lives; furthermore, we are also more willing, I believe, to consider trauma and circumstances such as cultural trauma. The experience of a collective group trauma has been more widely recognized since the death of so many Jewish people in the Holocaust was exposed. Over the past twenty years, we have finally begun to recognize the Holocaust that was of the Africanist people. However, there are those who do not believe that either event occurred. Since I believe that the African Holocaust was a definite event that caused immediate and long-term trauma to Africanist people, I can recognize the cultural trauma that has occurred as a result.

The following is an extract from the oral narrative of former slave Fanny Cannady about her early years in slavery:

> I don' 'member much 'bout de sojers an' de fightin' in de War den, kzae I wuzn' much more den six years ole at de Surrender, but I do 'member how Marse Jordan Moses shot Leonard Allen, one of his slaves. I ain't never forgot dat. My mammy an pappy, Silo an' Fanny Moss, belonged to Marse Jordan and Mis' Sally Moss. Dey had 'bout three hundred niggahs an' mos' of dem worked in de cotton fields. Marse Jordan wuz hard on his niggahs. He worked dem overtime an' didn' give dem enough to eat. Dey didn't have good clothes either an' dey shoes wuz make out of wood. He had 'bout a dozen niggahs dat didn' do nothin' else but make wooden shoes for de slaves. De chillum didn' have no shoes a-tall; dey went barefooted in de snow an' ice, same as 'twuz summertime. I never had no shoes on my feets 'twell I wuz pas' ten years ole, an' dat wuz after dem Yankees done sets us free. I wuz skeered of Marse Jordan, an' all of de grown niggahs wuz too, 'cept Leonard an' Burrus Allen .... I wuz sort of skeered of Mis' Sally, too.

When Marse Jordan wuzn' rroun' she was sweet an' kind, but when wuz roun', she wuz er 'yes, suh, yes, suh," woman. Everthin' he tole her to do she done. He made her slap Mammy one time, 'kaze when she passes his coffee she spilled some in he sauce.

Mis' Sally hit Mammy easy, but Marse Jordan say, "Hit her, Sally. Hit de black bitch like she 'zerve to be hit." Den Mis' Sally draw back her hand an' hit Mammy in de face, pow. Den she went back to her place at the table an' play like she eatin' her breakfas'. Den when Marse Jordan leave, she come in de kitchen an' put her arms round' Mammy an' cry, an' Mammy pat her on de back an' she cry, too. I loved Mis' Sally when Marse Jordan wuzn' round.

(Cited in Mellon, 1988, pp. 78–80)

This is a short part of a narrative of one slave's particular experience of slavery. Her entire story is worthy of being told because she was born into slavery which she endured for a few years, was freed and then came also to see the aftermath of slavery. Her words tell us of the authenticity of cultural trauma. They also tell us of fear. As we consider the five stages of grief, grieving and death for the African diaspora bound by slavery, we must also consider their fear. Kübler-Ross and Kessler speak of anticipatory grief—the expectation that grief will come to a loved one who is found to be terminally ill. I believe that individuals bound in slavery endured *anticipatory grief* as well as fear. I also believe that we can call this experience of life post-traumatic stress disorder for those descendants who survived actual bodily enslavement but who could not escape psychological imprisonment.

The emotional state of denial encompasses the realization that another will not be alive in the body any longer while having an expectation that the individual could be present again at any moment. It seems that this perpetual state of ambiguity would add to the psychological stress of slaves.

The conflict was not only in the denial and trauma of shock and numbness caused by the continuous circle of slave death which took place on a plantation, but also by a cultural belief that life continued through an ancestral lineage. The heavy reliance on spiritual beliefs that was so pronounced within the slave community, speaks to the recognition of religious beliefs that held life as a continuum. The death of the body, in Africanist thinking, is a release from present suffering and a return to an ancestral realm. Mary Gaffney, a former slave, recalls:

When a slave died, we just dug a hole in the ground, built a fence around it, and piled him in. No singing, no preaching or praying, ever took place during slavery time. Maser would say, "Well he was a pretty good Negro. Guess he will go to Heaven, all right." And that was about all there was to a Negro funeral, then. *We would not even shed a tear, because he was gone where there would not be any more slaves. That was all the slave thought about, then: Not being a slave. Because slavery time was hell.*

(Cited in Mellon, 1988, p. 41; emphasis added)

I would note that as time progressed, the ability to hold onto the original rites of passage and rituals became less influential. The decades and centuries of slavery succeeded in removing some of the ancestral lineage markers of African culture.

There is no doubt about this. However, in the acknowledgement of the power of mirror neurons for recollection of emotional states, there is also the possibility of remembrance of cultural facts and artifacts. This, I believe, is important for providing hope in the face of despair. In a model of Africanist thinking based on cultural trauma there would be little use for denial.

I believe that the centuries-long effect of slavery would have over time minimized disbelief or denial. The casualness of taking a slave's life was so commonplace as to not disavow death. Denial would have had little place in the consciousness of ancestors surrounded by the fact of such a commonality of slaves dying frequently at the whim of plantation owners and their overseers. With this as a consideration, denial as a major aspect of a cycle of an Africanist grieving process would be absent. In addition, a philosophical underpinning of Africanist consciousness intertwined death as a part of life. The binding of these two rites of passage, I do not believe, would have left the African psyche, no matter the number of years of slavery.

> One day Marse Gregory come home on er furlow. He think he look pretty wid his sword clankin' an his boots shinin'. He wuz er colonel, lootenent, er somethin'. He wuz struttin roun' de yard showin' off Leonard Allen say under his breath, "Look at dat goddman sojer. He fightin' to keep us niggahs from bein' free." 'Bout dat time Marse Jordan come up. He look at Leonard an' say "Wat yo' mumblin' 'bout?" Dat bit Leonard wuzn' skeered. He say, "I say, "look at dat goddamn sojer. He fightin' to keep us niggahs from bein' free!" Marse Jordan's face begun to swell. It turned so red sat de blook near 'bout bust out. He turned to Pappy an' tole him to go an' bring him his shotgun. When Pappy come back Mis' Sally come wid him. De tears quz streamin' down her face. She run up to Marse Jordan an' caught his arm. Old Marse flung her off an' took de gun from Pappy. He leveled it on Leonard an' tole him to pull his shirt open. Leonard opened his shirt and stood dere big as er black giant, sneerin' at Old Marse. Den Mis' Sally run up again an' stood 'tween dat gun an' Leonard. Den Old Marse let down de gun. He reached over an' sapped Mis' Sally down, den picked up de gun an' shot er hold in Leonard's ches' big as yo' fist. Den he took up Mis Sally an' toted her in de house. But I wuz so skeered dat I run an' hid in de stable loft, an' even wid my eyes shut I could see Leonard layin' on de groun' wid dat bloody hole in his ches' an' dat sneer on his black mouf. After dat, Leonard's brother Burrus hated Ole Marse wus'n er snake. Den one night he run away.
>
> *Fanny Cannady, former slave (Mellon, 1988, pp. 80–81)*

Anger is another stage in the grieving process. When I first began to consider Kübler-Ross's model of grief, I expected that I would be able to use if not all of the five stages, then certainly the emotional stages as she had defined them. However, during the course of writing this book, I have found that the grief and grieving process which I am attempting to define for the African diaspora as a result of slavery resists being captured within the frame of the Kübler-Ross model. It appears that the nature of the intergenerational trauma of slavery cannot be accounted for in a model that fails to include a view on racism, trauma or culture. I do, however, find that her contemporary frame may be considered appropriate for the way in which some of us might face grief today—without taking into account any cultural factors.

In thinking about the emotion of anger within the context of the loss of a partner, child or family member, anger finds its way into the body of the grieving Other who has been left behind. It seems that this must happen in order for the possibility of the final stage of acceptance to occur. In their discussion of anger Kübler-Ross and Kessler say, "Underneath anger is pain, your pain. It is natural to feel deserted and abandoned, but we live in a society that fears anger. People often tell us our anger is misplaced, inappropriate, or disproportionate" (2014, p. 15)

In Chapter 7 of this volume, I discuss grief as anger within the stereotype and archetype of the angry black woman so I will not expand on this topic within this chapter except to develop the idea of a deeply felt cultural anger that grows out of cultural trauma. Within the African diaspora, there continues to be a place for anger that covers grief.

One of the major aspects of American racism has been its reluctance to accept that descendants of slavery can still remain angry over the very *fact* of slavery. The racial facts of what has happened not only to them through Reconstruction, the history of Jim Crow segregation and lynching, but also to their ancestors, remains unresolved for many individuals of Africanist ancestry. I agree with Kübler-Ross and Kessler that there may be pain, an unspeakable pain, that underscores this anger. In the history of America, this does not want to be acknowledged or accepted. During the days of revolt in the 1960s, which gave rise to the Black Power movement and an expression of African American anger, there appeared to be a consistent refusal to create any space for black anger in the minds of white Americans—and even some black Americans. Some of this rage has gone back into the collective shadow. But not all of it and so today with the election of Donald Trump, we, as an American collective once again encounter the face of anger in the rise of white nationalism. Under the surface of Africanist collective conformity is the cultural trauma, which claims the archetypal DNA of former slaves. In the struggle for freedom and the continual ongoing fight for an empowered identity, African Americans hold onto and remember the archetypal event of American slavery.

The sometimes-overwhelming demand of the American collective during moments of heightened frustration, or white rage, will still not allow for any psychic space of black anger. The continued engagement at this level keeps a racial tension of "Opposites" in play that only appears to become resolved through laws. However, we know that the judicial system is not working in a racially ethical manner because of the disproportionately large number of African American men who are incarcerated.

It is my belief that because of this refusal to allow African Americans to feel their anger and grievance about slavery and racism, and the reluctance to accept a *consistently* recognized acknowledgement of the fact of slavery and also its aftermath, we as a collective remain on a merry-go-round of racial tensions, violence and eruptions.

The anger that covers pain in the grieving process is one that belongs to an African American culture that has never been able to find enough identity in an American psyche. The racism built into American life—every phase of it—has limited and exasperated attempts by the African diaspora to partake in and enjoy the fullness of American life. When confronted with this reality, some resist it declaring that African Americans have had as many equal opportunities as any others who have arrived on America's shores. This in itself is a fallacy due to the nature of the arrival of African Americans. They came as slaves and continued to experience the racist effects of slavery for centuries. Even in freedom, following the Civil War, until the present day, the intense work for civil liberties and the right to fully enjoy the pleasure of *being* psychologically, socially and financially embodied in America eludes many African Americans.

Though there are many African Americans who can claim financial success, racism can strip away dignity at a moment's notice. There is no security in America when one is of African ancestry. This is the lesson that African American children learn early in life. It is a lesson learned during slavery and is still relevant today.

African diaspora cultural trauma can reflect anger that may only appear to be extinguished. The broader collective does not wish to see this anger and has no place for it. The internal group struggle is to find a release for this anger, as well as a passage to the underlying grief and pain. The model inclusive of anger that I propose is one that overtly recognizes cultural trauma and includes grief at a culturally conscious level.

The third stage in the grief process is *bargaining*. This usually happens between the individual in grief who has lost a loved one and a spiritual being. In contemporary life this might be God. The desire to stay united with the loved one motivates the grieving individual towards a plea consisting of promises that cannot be realized because the loved one's death is inevitable.

In the case of African diaspora, bargaining had little effect on relieving the occurrence of death. The demands of the plantation system and the interlocking economic system of slavery, dependent on the lives of slaves, almost guaranteed that attempting to negotiate for continued life would be meaningless. African slaves had no means of bargaining for their lives with the men who had stolen them from Africa. Any real bargain had already been made between a local tribesman and white ship captains who would cross the Atlantic Ocean with a hold full of African people, soon to be American slaves if they survived the voyage.

Bargaining for one's own life or that of another had little effect within the non-responsive African trade system. Attempting to obtain salvation for the self or another was pointless in most cases. Most attempts at bargaining—whether with a slaver, ancestors or God—a Supreme Being—only appeared to intensify the likelihood of punishment or death.

> One day, in 'bout er week, Mis' Sally wuz feedin' de chickens when she heard somethin' in de polkberry bushes behin' de henhouse. She didn't go roun' de house but she went inside an' looked through de crack. Dere wuz Burrus layin' down in de bushes. He was near 'bout starved 'kaze he hadn't had nothin' to eat since he done run away.
>
> Mis' Sally whisper an' tole him to lay still, dat she goin' to slip him somethin' to eat …. Den, while she talk she take de pan an' go on to de chicken house, but Ole Marse he go, too. When dey got to de henhouse Ole Marse' puppy begun sniffin' roun'. … Den he foun' Burrus layin' in de polkberry bushes. Dey took Burrus to de whippin' post. Dey strip off his shirt. Den dey put his head an' hands through de holes in de top an' tied his feets to de bottom. Den Ole Marse took de whip. Dat lash hiss like col' water on er red hot iron when it come through de air, an' every time it hit Burrus it lef' er streak of blood. Time Ole Marse finish, Burrus back look like er piece of raw beef. Dey laid Burrus face down on er plank, den dey poured turpentine in all dem cut places. It burned like fire but dat niggah didn't know nothin' 'bout it, 'kaze he done passed out from pain. But, all his life dat black man toted dem scars on his back.
>
> *Fanny Cannady, former slave (Mellon, 1988, pp. 81–82)*

Fanny Cannady is a child birthed into slavery and released into freedom while still a child. In her narrative about her life, she says that she doesn't remember much about being freed before the Civil War but she seems to remember all of the painful events while held as a slave by slave owner Jordan. She especially remembers the death of Allen Leonard and the scars of Burrus. According to Cannady, Leonard does not bargain for his life. As was the case in many stories about slaves who tried to run away, Burrus has no choice but to return to the plantation. Attempts to get food and find safety without support proved futile for many slaves. They were forced to return to the plantation where they were severely beaten or killed. There are no places in slave narratives where bargaining is seen as an option for escaping death. Within a philosophical framework where death will give relief, it could be understood that Leonard would open his shirt, thereby almost demanding that death take him. Nowhere in the slavery system was there a place for bargaining though there are stories of family members begging to be allowed to stay together rather than separated at auction. Death and grief were key elements of slavery life. However, nowhere in this human system of death was bargaining for life generally rewarded.

This perhaps also shows the absence of compassion. In their discussion of depression Kübler-Ross and Kessler say, "After bargaining our attention moves squarely into the present. Empty feelings present themselves, and grief enters our lives on a deeper level than we ever imagined. This depressive stage feels as though it will last forever" (2014, p. 20). I would suggest that this depression does in fact *last forever*. I believe that this is the core expression of archetypal grief that presents itself in the clinical setting with most of my women patients of Africanist ancestry. The nature of slavery only rarely allowed for the belief that freedom was possible. Though during the days of the American Revolution and the following decade, the spirit of Enlightenment ideals which had fueled the American Revolution forced many Americans to free their slaves, the thrust at the beginning of the 1800s was to create laws which forbade freeing slaves. This was proposed not only to better serve the plantation system economically but also because there grew to be a much greater fear amongst plantation owners of slave revolts.

> Clearly most slaves were not passive, agreeable puppets who could be manipulated at will, though in every group such people probably exist. As human beings, most slaves had one overriding objective: self-preservation at a minimal cost of degradation and loss of self-respect. For most, the goal of "freedom" was simply unrealistic, especially after the sharp decline in manumissions, except under highly unusual circumstances.
> *(Davis, 2006, p. 195)*

Human, animal and plant life—none were meant to be captured and imprisoned. It is natural that depression would become a very significant experience for African American slaves. This experience would become "normalized" in the lives of slaves. Oftentimes, strategies were created by plantation owners to evoke a false happiness in slaves that did not exist and was not long-lasting. It was meant to replace the despair and depression of slaves.

> I mus' tell you 'bout dat whiskey and brandy. Massa have he own still and allus have three barrels or more whiskey and brandy on hand. Den, on Christmas Day, him puts a tub of whiskey or brandy in de yard and hangs tin cups round de tub. Us helps ourselves. At first, us start jokin' with each other. Den, us starts to sing and everybody am happy. Massa watches us, and if one us gittin' too much, Massa sends him to he cabin and he slept it off. Anyway, dat was one day on Mass's place when all am happy and forgets dey am slaves.
> *Charley Hurt, former slave (Mellon, 1988, p. 143)*

Depression is a lowering of the psychological ability to find any possibility for happiness in one's life. It is a state characterized by withdrawal and a disbelief that life is worth living or that change is possible to create a better, more joyful life. When considering the depression of which Kübler-Ross speaks during the healing process that follows the death of a loved one, there can be an understanding that this period of profound unhappiness will pass. The depression that comes as a result of the death of an individual might appear to last for several months, even a few years. When I reflect on depression as an emotional feature of slaves, I do not see a release from depression. It appears as a possible life experience that must be endured in order to survive.

If depression comes as a result of the loss of love, affection, psychological bonding with another, then this was the continuous cycle experienced by most Africanist individuals bound by slavery. One of the ultimate rationales given for slavery was that it did bring and keep people together.

This justification for slavery was articulated most recently by Roy Moore who in mid-2018 was running for election to the US Senate to replace the newly appointed Jeff Sessions. Moore has twice been removed from the Alabama Supreme Court in the wake of racist rulings. The recent campaign has been full of stories related by women claiming to have been sexually assaulted when they were teenagers. His political life as reported by the media indicates that he allegedly holds misogynistic and racist views. When he says that slavery thrived in the time when America was great—at her best—and references slavery times as these best of times because families were "together," we can see that we remain in almost the same societal quandary. American racism is alive and thriving in the consciousness of the American collective while black people continue to seek freedom in all of its many forms.

The justifications for slavery continued into the 21st century and are articulated by elected officials who believe in slavery having been a necessary aspect of American society. The emotional sadness and depression that might occur amongst the African diaspora is insignificant to them. The idea that these "families' who were bought and sold through the plantation system can be considered a positive aspect of American life due to slavery is appalling. That this kind of thinking should remain part of an American psyche probably reflects the views of people who may be inclined to vote for Moore.

The belief that slavery was good for us as Americans because it kept families together, and is what makes America great, is an irrational justification that holds no truth for the African diaspora nor for any other rationally thinking American. It is the voice of white supremacy.

"Clinical depression is a group of illnesses that may be characterized by a long-term or excessively depressed state" (Kübler-Ross and Kessler, 2014, p. 23). This is the kind of depression which I believe became an acquired part of the lives of my ancestors. Without the possibility of hope of freedom from slavery, the depression that probably set in upon being captured in Africa, took hold and was never really released from the African American psyche.

What is the consistent and frequent healing that would have supported a letting go of this type of depression? How have we as a cultural group begun to have enough of the conversations regarding group healing that this level of cultural trauma *can* heal? What would it take for such a beginning and engagement with healing to commence? These questions and others like them must be at the forefront of Africanist thinking in order for the aftermath of such a profound depression to become identified for what it is. We have been told for centuries that slavery required no healing or not much. White American guilt, in different ways, continues to carry on this story. We as Africanist people must find our own way to heal ourselves, and to create our own story derived from our own African consciousness. We must ask the question—what do we need in order to continue our post-slavery healing that has affected us as cultural trauma?

The last stage in Kübler-Ross and Kessler's conceptualization concerns the state of psychological *acceptance*.

> Acceptance is often confused with the notion of being all right or okay with what has happened. This is not the case. Most people don't ever feel okay or all right about the loss of a loved one. This stage is about accepting the reality that our loved one is physically gone and recognizing that this new reality is the permanent reality. *We will never like this reality or make it okay, but eventually we accept it.*
>
> *(2014, pp. 24–25; emphasis added)*

Within the context of an Africanist frame that presupposes accepting the death of loved one and believing that they will enter into the next phase of the afterlife, does not require much of a stretch of imagination. Oftentimes, it is not an acceptance based on the fact of the death of family members and ancestors but rather the circumstances of *how* they died. There was such a great loss due to the numbers who did not survive the crossing of the Atlantic Ocean.. This does not include those who perished once arriving at the North American continent.

> It is important to remember that in the beginning, African slaves were not taken to the Americas but rather to Iberia and the Atlantic islands. Brazil only began importing a significant number of black slaves in the late 1500s, approximately 140 years after they were first brought to Portugal. It took another century before the truly hemispheric slave trade began to rise to wholly new levels, peaking in the late eighteenth century. From 1700 to 1880 an estimated 9.47 million slaves were deported from Africa, or about 86.3 percent of the total transatlantic slave migration (not counting shipboard mortality). Yet as early as 1550 black slaves constituted 10 percent of Lisbon's population of about 1,000,000.
>
> *(Davis, 2006, p. 93)*

During the acceptance stage of grief, the still-living are beginning to release sorrow and anger. These emotions can be reoccurring, as there is no ongoing consistent pattern in which they will become evident in the grieving child, mother or daughter. However, I would propose that to those of the African diaspora affected by slavery and its aftermath, acceptance becomes a perpetual state of *we will never like this reality or make it okay* (Kübler-Ross and Kessler, 2014, pp. 24–25). I think it is acceptance in an essentially different way than that proposed by Kübler-Ross and Kessler.

This type of *acceptance* by the African diaspora travels through an Africanist consciousness that continues to demand acknowledgement and apology for not only the fact of slavery but also for the continuing racist aftermath that beleaguers us in the 21st century. It might be difficult to conceive of thousands of one's ancestors arriving in America in the hold of a slave ship. This fact alone would make one have a particular way in which to hold acceptance—it might be conditioned by centuries of psychic, archetypal energy. It might be difficult to conceive of thousands of one's ancestors being bought and sold at auction while white individuals became economically wealthy. Conceiving of this might allow descendants the freedom to feel into the agedness of never liking a selective reality that speaks to the deaths of so many—kin and non-kin alike.

The inability to *make it okay*—the acceptance of such cultural trauma—highlights the difference between a model of grief suited to those without such cultural trauma and those held in such a psychological prison. The African diaspora has suffered through generations of making many things of great emotional pain *okay*. Joy DeGruy, author of *Post Traumatic Slave Syndrome: America's Legacy of Enduring Injury and Healing* states:

> The racist socialization of African Americans began with slavery and continued throughout American history. Whites have consistently been portrayed and perceived as superior, powerful and right. For those who were educated and could read, book after book asserted that blacks, as well as other peoples of color, were dirty, lustful, stupid, immoral, incapable of reasoning .... inferior to whites in every way.
>
> As movies became popular the early 20th century, blacks were consistently cast in the roles of servants and buffoons. Little changed with the advent of radio and later television. It was the rare exception when a black character was portrayed as a dignified, competent and caring human being.
>
> *(2005, p. 137)*

As previously stated, I had an idea that the five stages of grief would somehow provide a steady, solid possible frame for seeing more deeply into the grieving process of those members of the Africanist popular affected by the cultural trauma of slavery. I have much appreciation for this model within the close intimate clinical work with patients. However, as I attempted to extrapolate this theory of death and grieving, it did not seem expansive enough to hold those who had suffered such cultural trauma—a holocaust—caused by racism. The genocide movement against Africanist people through the period of enslavement and afterwards during segregation, does not fold so easily into a theory formulated for many but without the consideration of racism as a factor.

I believe that one's grief, anger and acceptance of dying and death belongs within the context of one's ethnic background and cultural consciousness.

Stages of grief can reflect the Africanist idea that acceptance is as viably possible as is death.

American slavery makes this impossible. Acceptance matched with the peculiarity of an American society still refusing to accept the cruel history of slavery and its racist legacy, leaves much to be processed, held in reflection, and ways found for reparation..

7

GRIEF AS ANGER

Hidden grief

We frequently believe that we can understand all the pain and emotional suffering endured during a lifetime by another. I remember when my mother's first cousin lost her young son in a summer river swimming accident. My mother kept saying, "It's the saddest thing." I believe she had witnessed much to make her extremely sad in her lifetime. Her sadness and the way in which she was strong—always fighting a current of abuse at home—made her seem invincible. As time has progressed, I have come to realize that I may have understood only a very small amount of my own mother's suffering. Many of my reference points are what she would not allow me to do at home or be because she had already experienced the underbelly of such an existence. Most of her grief remained hidden from me, and even when she was angry, her anger could appear only as some form of sadness.

Slavery's legacy includes the ongoing stigmatization of Africanist women as angry, disagreeable and malcontented. If we are not seen in this way, then we are identified as whores, always available sexually, and intentionally promiscuous. This latter colonizing collective image is much easier to understand that the former. One of the main purposes of slavery, the economic reign over property—human beings—was maintained through the use of control. Even from the early days of slavery African women began to experience this control as it was displayed on slave ships.

> Male and female slavery was different from the very beginning. As noted previously, women didn't generally travel the middle passage in the holds of slave ships but took the dreaded journey on the quarter deck. According to the 1789 Report of the Committee of the Privy Council, the female passage was further distinguished from that of males in that women and girls were not shackled .... This policy had at least two significant consequences for black

women. First, they were more easily accessible to the criminal whims and sexual desires of seamen, and few attempts were made to keep the crew members of slave ships from molesting African women. As one slaver reported, officers were permitted to indulge their passions at pleasure and were "sometimes guilty of such brutal excesses as disgrace human nature."

(White, 1998, p. 63)

In *Inhuman Bondage* David Brion Davis described the Portuguese transportation of female slaves in the 1500s: "A major motive for separating the women was the fear that they would encourage the males to revolt (but the separation of sexes also made it far easier for members of the crew to rape black women, a very common occurrence)" (2006, p. 93).

This particular type of brutality exercised against African women continued throughout all the centuries of slavery. It changed its form during different historical periods but never really ceased. The most obviously famous case of such a display of the control and power of white men over Africanist women was Thomas Jefferson and his never-ending relationship with his slave-mistress. The descendants of this relationship are alive today and given voice to their ancestral inheritance as descendants of a former president of the United States, slave owner and a mother slave. This example shows the complexity of American racial relations. Jefferson refused to relinquish his relationship with his slave through all the years of his marriage to a white woman.

He also never freed his slaves. This is the type of condition under which Africanist women lived. The difficulty of maintaining personal dignity in an American society that supported racism, while the collective remained ambivalent about slavery, was an immense psychological burden for African American women.

In *When and Where I Enter: The Impact of Black Women on Race and Sex in America* Paula Giddings discusses the "new slavery" which began to take place in America from 1830 onward due to the intensification of the Abolitionist movement and the increase in the number of slaves living on Southern plantation. Threatened by the Nat Turner revolt, whites began to consider ways in which to treat their slaves *more humanely*. The word "domesticated" became more common and affected African American women in a way that was consistent with the continued control of them through white male sexualized behavior.

> The Victorian "extended" family also put the "moral" categories of women into sharp relief. The White wife was hoisted on a pedestal so high that she was beyond the sensual reach of her own husband. Black women were consigned to the other end of the scale, as mistresses, whores, or breeders.
>
> *(1988, p. 43)*

Historical evidence regarding the social and psychological projections placed on Africanist women as unworthy beings has a very long history. Women were not only subjected to rape but also to whippings and beatings just as any slave man or child would have been. This physical abuse could come at any time for any reason. The following is from Jacqueline Jones in *Labor of Love, Labor of Sorrow: Black Women, Work and the Family from Slavery to the Present*.

> For most enslaved domestics, housework involved hard, steady, often strenuous labor as they juggled the demands made by the mistress and other members of the master's family. Mingo White of Alabama never forgot that his mother had shouldered a workload "too heavy for any one person." She served as personal maid to the master's daughter, cooked for all the hands on the plantation, carded cotton, spun a daily quota of thread, and wove and dyed cloth. Every Wednesday she carried the white family's laundry three-quarters of a mile to a creek, where she beat each garment with a wooden paddle. Ironing consumed the rest of her day. Like the lowliest field-hand, she felt the lash if any tasks went undone.
>
> *(2010, p. 21)*

When we read the close details of the life of slaves we can barely imagine this life. Yet this was the life of millions of African diaspora female ancestors who provided the economic wealth for white Americans. African American women became known as angry, rage-filled malcontents. How did we come to be known in this way? What is hidden beneath this image, stereotype and almost archetypal pattern of the *angry black woman*? If we hold the life experiences of an African American slave woman mirrored against what might be expected of her emotionally, what might we see?

I believe that a challenge of allowing this mothering slave woman to have *any* feelings is because as a controlled entity of another she was prohibited from being able to truly express her own desires or wishes. An absolute fact of slavery for both black adult men and women was the restriction on what was allowed to be spoken—especially to whites, be they white children or adults. Given this factor in most black-white slavery relationships, where would one anticipate the emotions of a slave would escape to? Blacks were restricted to speaking with one another in each other's company—not necessarily in the presence of any whites. This also proved best for slaves as they could protect themselves from the slave owner knowing what their thoughts might be.

Fanny Cannady, a former slave, tells us that she witnessed Leonard being shot dead after speaking his mind to Jordan, the slave owner. In this narrative, we can almost forget the young Fanny who bears witness to this murder. Now I can say murder. For centuries Africanist people were not permitted to voice their protest against the deaths of fellow African lineage people. These deaths were justified by white Christian religion, philosophy or "science." Chained and manacled, working under the whip—these were not conditions conducive to open verbal rebellion. It took time for Africanist people to develop this ability and to move from chained human beings to people who would take action against being chained. The physical geography of the land also played a large part in this gaining of freedom.

Africanist people in countries such as Haiti were freed much earlier than were African Americans.

I can ask what the effect would be on this child, Fanny Cannady, who lived in slavery and moved to freedom. How many children in slavery would bear witness to murder and physical violence over the centuries? Might we say every slave child? How would these experiences affect the psychology of these children? What influence have mirror neurons played in the intergenerational cognitive development of mother to child?

Slaves could have feelings when they were given permission to have these feelings—the location and time were determined by the slave owners. The expression of ideas, emotions or dislikes was usually forbidden unless expressly demanded by the "master." Another justification for slavery was that Africans and later African Americans were incapable of having ideas and certainly did not know what they wanted because they could not think and therefore deserved to be silent unless given permission to speak.

This selective idea that Africanist people were incapable of thinking came to America not just through seamen, but also via the work of missionaries and anthropologists who had traveled to Africa attempting to validate or research their own racial theories. One of the most popular books of its time for many decades was *How Natives Think* (Levy-Bruhl, 1960).

> The main thesis of Levy-Bruhl's theory (1960) was that indigenous people formed a collective representation held together by a group experience of symbols. These symbols were both internal and external. Levy-Bruhl (1960) proposed that this collective included myths and rituals that determined how group members would behave. According to Levy-Bruhl (1960), indigenous people were controlled by their senses and emotions, not their ability to reason. Eventually, Levy-Bruhl replaced the term "pre-logical" with "logic and mystical" though this in no way changed his basic belief about African people's ability to reason. In a manner similar to Sigmund Freud's, Levy-Bruhl (1960) wrote in part to counter the influence of rationalism in European society. The latter's emphasis on finding a community of individuals whom Europeans could emulate for their "emotionalism" was readily welcomed in the early years of the 20th century.
>
> (Brewster, 2011, p. 84)

The irrational creation of the idea of extreme "emotionalism" in Africans became a convoluted narrative that held them as both without reason and bearers only of emotions. Would this have been a possible reason for the limitations placed on Africans talking and developing English-speaking skills? How afraid were colonizing whites of the possible emotional states of Africans? Could this lead to revolts against slavery? The focused attention of whites to prevent Africans from learning English and from speaking to one another certainly suggests an irrational fear against African "emotionalism." During the period following Reconstruction and

72 Grief as anger

at the turn of the 19th century, the character of "Sambo" developed into a Vaudeville clown—initially played by white men imitating black men. The image of the black man as a buffoon was carried over into the early days of film. Such imagery reinforced at a visual level the lack of intelligence of black men.

The idea and later theory of the lack of intellectual functioning of Africans found its way into the basic theoretical structure of Jung's analytical psychology, the field of American psychology most often based on theories of eugenics.

The silencing of Africanist people was attempted and in different ways was successful. As time passed, as Africanist people became more fluent in the language of oppression, they began to find ways of speaking for themselves. The expression of feelings against racism initially came through those in the South who revolted against their imprisonment of slavery. Words followed. Running away and revolts came later.

> When Dr. Cannon found out dat his carriage driver had larned to read and write whilst he was takin' de doctor's chillum to and f'om school, he had dat nigger's thumbs cut off, and put another boy to doin de drivin in his place.
> *Tom Hawkins, former slave (Cited in Mellon, 1988, p. 198)*

During the slavery era, Africanist women had ways of expressing their feelings but these were seldom respected. However, the need for expression was strong and should have been expected. Punishment for speaking out could be minimal or severe.

> My mother, she didn't work in the field. She worked at a loom. She worked so long and so often that once she went to sleep at the loom. Her master's boy saw her and told his mother. His mother told him to take a whip and wear her out. He took a stick and went out to beat her awake. He beat my mother till she woke up. When she woke up, she took a pole out of the loom and beat him nearly to death with it. He hollered, "Don't beat me no more, and I won't let 'em whip you." She said, "I'm goin' to kill you. These black titties sucked you, and then you come out here to beat me." And when she left him, he wasn't able to walk. And that was the last I seen of her until after Freedom. She went out and got an old cow that she used to milk—Dolly, she called it. She rode away from the plantation, because she knew they would kill her, if she stayed.
> *Ellen Cragin, former slave (Cited in Mellon, 1988, pp. 236–238)*

My retelling of the lives of Africanist women slaves and former slaves is in service of them having a story that *can* validated as true as well as imagined. The imagination at work in this way allows for belief to take place. There has been a different historical story told by many over the centuries who claim that Africanist history is dead. The story of the lives of those who came across the Atlantic is dead and gone—nothing to talk about now, forget it. I disagree with this. The shaping of our African American consciousness is due to the experiences of our ancestors who came through the Middle Passage as well as those who never left Africa. There is a way in which we can be taught to give up holding that psychic place of *emptiness* for those who perished. I believe that we are charged with filling this space with remembrance and sacredness for these ancestors. A part of the false history of African Americans is that we really had no past except the non-truth one reported in white history books that were written without our voices. Each and every time we have an opportunity to refute this falsehood we must do so. We do not worship our ancestors. We honor them.

The African American cultural complex

Jungian analyst Samuel Kimbles in *Phantom Narratives: The Unseen Contributions to Psyche* relates the following dream:

> In the first dream, which I had the night before my interview for admission to the analytic training program in San Francisco, I found myself waiting for the Admissions Committee (of the analytic training institute) to call me for my interview. I was sitting with a number of other black men in a mosque of some sort. They were all dressed in black suits. Someone on the Admissions Committee then called my name. I got up, and as I was about to leave the room in which I had been waiting, the door was barred by several of the black men. They said they would not let me pass until I demonstrated to them our secret handshake. My giving them the sign of this handshake would let them know that I would never forget them.
>
> *(2014, p. 4)*

A portion of the author's interpretation of this dream would seem to indicate that the group would be important to his training. In fact, he says, "That was the promise I made by giving the handshake that signified I would not forget the group. Kinship and loyalty issues, power dynamics, oppression, and guilt could, therefore, remain in my mind as a context for analytic training" (ibid., p. 5).

Kimbles' work focuses on the cultural complexes. His definition of these complexs has several basis ideas. I believe it is important to name these complexes as Kimbles himself has done:

1. Cultural complexes operate through the group's expectations, its definition of itself, its destiny, and its sense of its uniqueness. They operate through the group's fears, its enemies, and its attitudes toward other groups.
2. Cultural complexes are a dynamic system of relations that serve the basic need for belonging and identity through linking personal experiences and group expectations as these are mediated by ethnicity, race, religion, and gender processes.
3. Cultural complexes impose constraints on the perception of differences or accentuate them, emphasize identification with the group or differentiation

from the group, and allow for feelings of belonging to or being alienated from the group.
4. Cultural complexes allow us to relate psychologically to cultural factors that operate beyond the individual but intersect with the individual's sense of self.
5. Cultural complexes are the psyche's way of narrating its relationship to the group. *(2014, pp. 5–6)*

Kimbles' theoretical concept of the cultural complex brings into focus a primary idea that a cultural complex is for the group as well as for individual functioning within a group. In deepening his concept regarding the cultural complex, Kimbles states:

> In short, if the personal unconscious can be understood through personal complexes, the cultural unconscious can be understood through cultural complexes. Both personal and cultural complexes arise out of archetypal aspects of the psyche and provide affect, image, structure, and dynamism to individual and group life. Cultural complexes function between the personal and archetypal psyche by linking the two realms in group and individual life.
>
> *(2014, p. 68)*

African Americans are situated within a cultural complex that holds not only the positive images and dynamism of their individual lives but also that of the group. This group dynamic also contains the phantoms of the past lives of those who have preceded them. The connection between those who have passed into death and those who remain are connected at an archetypal level that brings into a cultural reality the soul of the group.

When present-day Africanist mothers fear for the safety of their children I believe they are seeing and recognizing the phantoms of mothering slaves. These reflective *unseen phantoms* linger and help to form an essential aspect of this group. The fear of physical danger that can create an invisible field—threads running through the group, a cultural complex, reminiscent of the fear of running away from a plantation and being chased by dogs and a slave owner. As we remember the history of our ancestors, it would seem likely that the phantom energy of their suffering and emotional trauma become constellated in our consciousness. The emotions of this constellation can show themselves in any number of ways. The iconic image of angry black women forms and rises into the personal unconscious.

Angry black woman

One of the most relevant aspects of Jungian psychology is its willingness, even an actual desire, to go into the darkness. I'm not referring to the sociological placement of a negative *nigredo* onto Africanist people with all of its racist history. I'm referring to the darkness that can make us afraid of pursuing a truth that lives in that unconscious place that causes us to have nightmares. This is the location where we cannot hide individual truths nor what belongs to a particular group of people based on cultural complexes with all of their projections, anxieties and possible rage at the Other.

I believe that the angry black woman stereotype is like any other that developed in the American psyche. When a stereotype becomes formed in the American collective and is related to ethnicity and racism we must search hard to find the kernel of truth concealed by collective shadow. Our work as psychological beings is to move through layers of consciousness finding nuances and the essence of who we are and what belongs to us as members of a particular cultural group.

In this chapter I have revisited stories of the Africanist experience under American slavery. These are not narratives that are easy to bear—they are not meant to be because they represent an American truth that even today remains underreported and in many situations unwanted. This is part of the ongoing struggle of the history of racial relations in America.

A willingness on the part of American Jungians to enter into discussions about racism contained in some Jungian theories is beginning to emerge. With this emergence must come the shadowed part of the African American experience which included them as research subjects and racial victims of American psychology. This would include Jungian psychology (Brewster, 2017). One of our struggles as Americans attempting to resolve issues of racism is that we continue to try to escape into the shadows of racism by ignoring our cultural and racial complexes. We will desire to join and be with others in our "tribe" in kinship. This is how we are meant to be—connected through memory, blood and ancestral lineage. There is no reason why Africanist people should try to hide or feel shame for their collective past. A pronounced element of racism is a projection onto the Other is that they have done "something" wrong. In the case of American racism it is that African Americans are wrong by their very existence in America. As W. E. Dubois and many others have recognized, they have been designated as the "problem" in American society.

When I reflect on the angry black woman symbol I recognize her creation as evolving from different points on the horizon of racial consciousness and complexes. The first point of recognition is from the historical heritage of how Africanist women have arrived and lived in America since first being brought here as slaves. The instances of them being raped on voyages across the Atlantic Ocean are facts. Facts we may not wish to take note of, but our contemporary denial still cannot erase these facts. We must remember that this is a circumstance that lasted for centuries.

The attempts to erase these historical facts are part of a racism that wishes to create a cover of invisibility around a past that we must first *see* in order to heal. We may not have always known about the frequency of African women being raped on Middle Passage voyages but we know of this same sexual assault occurring on plantations and white households in America. The history of the Africanist woman includes sexual and physical abuse at the beginning of slavery and throughout her American life. In *At the Dark End of the Street: Black Women, Rape and Resistance*, Danielle L. McGuire recounts part of the judicial history of African American women seeking justice after being raped:

> In the 1940s it was nearly impossible for black victims of sexualized violence to receive justice in the courts. In 1944 a grand jury in Henry County, Alabama, refused to indict Recy Taylor's assailants despite their admissions, a gubernatorial intervention, and a national campaign for her defense. In 1949 the Montgomery police department would not even hold a lineup for Gertrude Perkins, who charged two officers with kidnapping and rape. After a citywide protest, Perkins had her day in court, but the grand jury refused to indict anyone for the crime. Black women had achieved small victories in their fight for bodily integrity throughout the 1950s, but they were few and far between. It was not until 1959 that an all-white jury in Tallahassee, Florida, sentenced four white men to prison for life in the brutal gang rape of Betty Jean Owens. It took another six years before Mississippi, the most unreconstructed Southern state, followed suit. In 1965 an all-white jury in Hattiesburg sent Norman Cannon to prison for life for kidnapping and raping Rosa Lee Coates. Victories of the mid-1960s rested on decades of black women's organizing and personal testimony …. In 1974 Joan Little became the symbol of a campaign to defend black womanhood and to call attention to the sexualized racial violence that still existed ten years after Congress passed the 1965 Voting Rights Act.
>
> *(2011, p. 248)*

In relating a little of the history of the struggle of African American women to find justice in the court system, I return to the concept of the angry black woman. A stereotype contains some element of truth. As the mythology, symbolism, iconic popularity of the angry black woman grew perhaps there have not been enough words addressing the depth of this "representation" of the Africanist female. As we have seen throughout this writing, history and oral stories, there has been a racist history of sexually assaulting black women with an unconscious general acceptance—with few exceptions—from the American collective since the time of slavery. Does this not make you angry?

The reluctance to see and understand why and how Africanist people can be angry dates back to the creation of a myth that claims that they had/have no right to be angry only assumes a false story that says that slavery was good because they were fed, clothed and housed. The refusal to accept that torturing, lynching and raping black women does not merit identification of a failure in the American collective only makes anger a more likely cultural group and an individual response.

From its earliest inception American society claimed it for "whites only." This sentiment could be found in the first political paper—the Constitution—establishing America as an independent country. It is not surprising then that racism has become a major force in the voices of white supremacy—those who want to make

America great again—before the Tenth Amendment. This is an old cry—to return Africans to Africa. Now *that* ship has certainly sailed. There is no going back because Africans and their descendants built this country through plantations, railroads, architecture and all the other ways that have created an American infrastructure. We cannot go back to pre-colonial days and will not go back to colonializing ones.

The cultural trauma of millions of Americans due to slavery is a very real circumstance. A key aspect of this cultural trauma has been the sexual assault of Africanist women. We can no longer hide this part of the American story. It took a very, very long time to bring it into the light. Now that it is there, it must remain.

Elisabeth Kübler-Ross understood that death necessitated a grieving process that included anger. This anger took place in the dying person as well as in those who would be left behind after the death of this individual. African Americans are part of a cultural collective that includes mother, grandmother, daughter, sister, aunt, cousin—the full matriarchal line of the feminine. All these women were and are affected by the cultural trauma of slavery. They are all still in an ancestral swell that sees through attempts to "forget" the abuse they have experienced through the phantom narratives of those who have gone before. When the proposition is put forward that it is time to move on and forget about the brutal sexual history of the treatment of Africanist women, the response to such a call must be that of other holocaust survivors—we must never forget. African American women are descendants of holocaust survivors. Genocidal physical and soul death ravaged this cultural collective for centuries. Anger is a most valuable emotional reaction because we are barely beginning to see any light of acknowledgement shine on this Africanist death of body, mind and soul. This emotion of anger belongs in a mirroring position for reflection on all that has come to pass in terms of the sexual abuse of black women. First we must remember, then we can heal. We can no longer permit our emotional bodies to be defined by those who wish to avoid their own cultural complexes.

In accepting the psychological reasons for even the existence of the initial emergence of an angry black woman construct, we know that this symbol holds the projection of others. We also know that within this projection is the anger and guilt of the Other. The idea of an angry black woman exists because there are many historical reasons forming the basis of causation for a profound anger.

What about the grief that lies beneath the anger? Can this be a consideration for a better psychological understanding of African American women? The strength of the black woman has also been mythologized. There is absolutely no doubt that the physical burden of Africanist slave women and their descendants was a heavy one. The descriptions that we have read of what plantation life was like for black women leaves us in no doubt about the emotional and physical strength that was required to stay alive. This does not take into account the psychological stress of living under the conditions of slavery. Grief as part of this stress was a normal part of any life.

When we work in the clinical setting, we most oftentimes realize that grief and sadness are beneath anger and rage. It may take time to get through the anger. It is not getting past it but rather studying and learning about the anger. It is making anger an acceptable part of the psyche. The same is true for your guilt. When death is involved I too believe as did Kübler-Ross and Kessler that we will go through periods, stages of grieving and that one of these will be anger. I also believe that for the African American woman, grief is oftentimes expressed as anger. It is my hope that as we consider the angry black woman we are also able to reflect on the emotional and tortuous ancestral memories that can be brought forward into the present day through a phantom narrative, an archetypal predisposition. We can understand our anger but what happens to the emotion of generations of former slaves? Jung says that our history is in our blood. The DNA that we live with identifies us as historical and archetypal human beings. If I feel into how my ancestors before me lived, whether through mirror neurons or the spirit of ancestors, how do I carry the traumatic emotions such as anger and the underlying grief of centuries-old slavery? I think that we could be angry but we must also hold a deep place for grief. So, when I hear about the angry black woman, I am also trying to hold psychic space for the grief-filled woman. Where does this grief emerge from and where does it go? I think that at this point it could be just enough to consider that such a thing exists—an underlying grief that rests within the bosoms of generations of African diaspora women. This grief can show itself as anger. Why not? Within the clinical setting oftentimes the emotion of anger covers sadness and sorrow. What would make this unlikely in a cultural collective that has survived 400 years of slavery? These are questions that I ask myself because of the American life that I lead—both personally and professionally. When we look deeply into the details of American slavery we can feel the nuances of suffering that must have lived in a field of human pain during those times. Anne C. Bailey, in *The Weeping Time: Memory and the Largest Slave Auction in American History*, explores the history of the slave-owning Butler family, the history of the Butler plantations on the Georgia Sea Islands, and the post-slavery experiences of the African Americans auctioned from Butler's plantation in March 1859. "It was the largest recorded slave auction in US history, advertised for weeks in newspapers and magazines across the country" (2017, p. 3).

In her description of the sale of one family, Bailey offers this historical narrative:

> Unfortunately, though the circumstances were similar, there was to be no such reprieve for Primus, Chattel no. 72, and Daphney, Chattel no. 73, a girl of three years, and a baby, Chattel no. 75, only one month old, that Daphney was holding protectively in her arms beneath a large shawl. This simple act of maternal love provoked the most boisterous remarks:
>
> "What do you keep your nigger covered up for? Pull off her blanket."
>
> "What's the matter with that gal" said another. "Has she got a headache?"
>
> "Who's going to bid on that nigger if you keep her covered up?" asked still another without regard for her newborn that had been born on Valentine's Day. "Let's see her face!"

Auctioneer Walsh had to repeatedly assure the boisterous buyers that there was no attempt at subterfuge: she was not an ill slave that they were trying to palm off as a healthy one but that Daphney had given birth only fifteen days before. For that, she was entitled to the "slight indulgence" of a shawl to wrap around her and her newborn baby to ward off the cold and the rain. With these assurances made, the bidding began and in the end Primus, who was a plantation carpenter, and Daphney, a rice hand, were both sold for $635. Their two small children, including the infant born on Valentine's Day, were also sold for the sum of $635 each.

(2017, p. 15)

The racial complex and African American women

If we consider the racial complex as a part of a cultural complex of African American women, there might just be a place for anger when we look at the historical treatment of black women in America. Why do we not include grief for these same women? Complexes are emotionally toned psychic responses to a trigger in the environment. The continuous, ever-ready projection that black women are aggressive or angry only makes them so. It becomes a circle of frustration and increased anger for the projector as well as the recipient of the projection. When the person projects this anger onto the Africanist woman, it is usually done without compassion. The perceived belief that the black woman is angry takes all responsibility for reclaiming this projection away from the white Other.

It is interesting to note that only since the last two presidential elections has the collective begun to speak more of a white rage or anger. Now we hear more often how white men are angry and feeling left out of the political and economic systems. Why are we as a society so committed to constantly discussing black women as being angry when we have just begun to scratch the surface of white anger in terms of discussing it? Was their willingness to treat Africanist people as chattels only borne out of economic greed, or was it not closely tied to their own rage? What of this rage?

> The truth is, white rage has undermined democracy, warped the Constitution, weakened the nation's ability to compete economically, squandered billions of dollars on baseless incarceration, rendered an entire region sick, poor, and woefully undereducated, and left cities nothing less than decimated.
>
> *(Anderson, 2017, p. 6)*

What are white people angry about? Is it simply a display of their own emotionally charged constellated racial complexes? A second point of recognition of the origin of the angry black woman narrative on a human landscape is a societal frame which in Jungian terms always sets you up to be an Opposite. This Opposite Other of the black woman exists across a historical landscape and is still an acceptable model of the first order—the white woman. I am not the first and will certainly not be the last African American writer who notes the paradigm that was established centuries ago putting the black woman at the bottom of a feminine hierarchy. This book is not a personal attack on the white woman, merely a review of how the black woman can be perceived as aggressive, uncouth and ignorant while the white woman remains the exact opposite.

Deborah Gray White notes the following in *Ar'n't I a Woman? Female Slaves in the Plantation South*:

> Black men and women were thought to have such insatiable sexual appetites that they had to go beyond the boundaries of their race to get satisfaction. It was black women who, many claimed, tempted men of the superior caste. White men, it was argued, never had to use authority or violence to obtain compliance from bonded women because the latter's morals were so relaxed. Proponents of this line of reasoning actually celebrated the societal stratification that made black women available but put white women out of reach. Northerners, they argued, debased the civilized; they defamed the white prostitute, cut her off from the hope of useful and profitable employment, immured her in a state of depravity. By contrast, Southern white women were kept free and pure from the taint of immorality because black women acted as a buffer against their degradation.
>
> *(1998, pp. 38–39)*

The myth of an unattractive black female—except when used for the physical pleasure of white men, had its beginnings in slavery. Initially, in the very early days of colonial America white women were used as breeders of children and as a means of enticing more black men onto the plantations. Over time, the laws changed and the "mixing of races" was forbidden. White women became elevated by the new social mores of the day. Due to the conditions of slavery black women were expected to remove their clothes on demand, be sexually assaulted and to serve as mistresses, and because of this black women became the female Other to white women. Black women were forced through the demands of slavery's racism to do and be all that white women were no longer allowed or expected to be. The evolution of this circumstance is discussed by Deborah Gray White in *Ar'n't I a Woman*:

> The idea that black women were exceptionally sensual first gained credence when Englishmen went to Africa to buy slaves. Unaccustomed to the requirements of a tropical climate, Europeans mistook semi-nudity for lewdness. Similarly, they misinterpreted African cultural traditions, so that polygamy was attributed to the Africans' uncontrolled lust, tribal dances were reduced to the level of orgy, and African religions lost the sacredness that had sustained generations of ancestral worshippers.
>
> *(1988: p. 29)*

It did not matter that a black female was still a girl-child—only just entering puberty—or a married woman committed to her husband, they had no choice but to do the bidding of the plantation owner or slave ship captain at a singular level and by American society at the collective one.

Racial complexes cause us to fall into the shadowed space of an archetypal possession that can demean the Other and lead to genocide of the cultural group of Other. The group experience of African Americans contains an ancestral legacy that includes the African Holocaust.

The women who birthed children into the plantation system would most certainly have felt anxiety, terror and anger at witnessing the deterioration of their African customs. Sacred rituals are for the maintenance of the community. Some survived the Middle Passage while others did not. The loss of so much because of this passage, unlike any that Africans had experienced before, would create profound grief covered by repressed anger. When we think about the symbolic angry black women, we are also required to remember some piece of the fabric of slavery's quilted archetypal memory transmitted intergenerationally. We must remember what this Africanist female carries unseen in her archetypal DNA—what she brings represents ancestral generations. Anger is her privilege and right, claimed through the generations of grief she has had to carry.

8
ARCHETYPAL GRIEF

> But Madam, let your grief be laid aside
> And let the fountain of your tears be dry'd;
> In vain they flow to wet the dusty plain,
> Your sighs are wasted to the skies in vain,
> Your pains they witness, but they can no more,
> While Death reigns tyrant o'er this mortal shore.
> *Phyllis Wheatley 1753–1784*

Marie Jenkins Schwartz states in *Birthing a Slave: Motherhood and Medicine in the Antebellum South*:

> As of 1808, when Congress ended the nation's participation in the international slave trade, planters could no longer import additional slaves from Africa or the West Indies: the only practical way of increasing the number of slave laborers was through new births. If enslaved mothers did not bear sufficient numbers of children to take the place of aged and dying workers, the south could not continue as a slave society.
>
> *(2009, p. 13)*

It is difficult to comprehend the sheer number of children who may have died during the voyage through the Middle Passage and in American slavery. We do know that the mortality rate of African American children in slavery was twice as high as that of white children. We also know that at least half of all Africanist infants died in the first year of life. These deaths were usually due to undernourishment or dysentery. It is suggested that in total between 30 million and 60 million Africanist people died while in slavery.

When I write of the death of Africanist children, I do not mean just death of the physical body but also that of the minds and emotional hearts of those children born into slavery and remaining so until their deaths as adults. I include those born into slavery and who lived to see freedom through the Emancipation Proclamation.

In Jungian psychology when one dreams of a child or children it is suggestive of the life potential and yet unrealized energy of the dreamer taking form in the image of the child. There is an indication of the direction the ego can take in reaching towards a desired wish or goal. In looking at the lost lives of Africanist children to the effects of slavery, we recognize how these children were never able to live to achieve their potential.

Both the physical and emotional deaths of children deprived the African diaspora of millions of individuals who could have helped to infuse the cultural consciousness with the necessary creative energy supportive of overall life enhancement. The negative energy drain of slavery took away from each generation the positive potential of unrealized expressions of a good energy that would have benefited not only the individual child but also the entire Africanist collective.

The powerful residual effects of American slavery have caused deep harm to every generation since the first African child was stolen. This fact does not negate the strength and monumental efforts and results of all the African diaspora who lived out their minimal lives bearing not only sorrow but also hope during slavery's darkest days. We must recognize not only the strength of what it took to survive those dark days but now that we have the strength we can view from a 21st-century perspective the deep centuries-long harm done by slavery to our forebears and their descendants.

We as a cultural collective do not have the privilege of casting aside knowledge or logic in our attempts to further deepen our understanding of the collective suffering we have experienced. Nor can we let ourselves be erased from history in service of repression of our collective memory. The recognition of harm done to us can move us from grievous to grief so that we may truly understand the depth of our suffering and anger. We acknowledge the grievous harm done. We intend to heal through authentic grief that will also last through future generations. The backward glance into the collective past is in remembrance and honor of those who suffered so that we might live, while holding vision and care for those to come.

If I am to believe in the archetypal presence of an energy within and outside of my unconscious self then I am willing to see the potential for changing consciousness to a more life-enhancing experience for Africanist people. I think that this begins with understanding, caring for and knowing our past. This obligation of caring for our culture is important especially because we continue to fight for it even as I write now in the 21st century.

Six generations ago my ancestors threw rice into the furrows of plantation land and picked cotton in fields cleared by *their* ancestors. When I speak of privilege and the claiming of the cultural past, it is deeply personal and I do this without any "scientific" apology for holding on to this past. It has taken many from each of my generational ancestral lineage to have those of us who live today, actually be alive today. It can only be a privilege to welcome a cultural past that continues to live in consciousness of myself as well as my cultural collective. As Africanist people we still must fight politically and socially within the American collective to be seen, respected and recognized as human beings. Our struggle continues. This struggle must reflect our damaged past. It will allow us to continue developing a healing perspective for our future. The spirits of those children lost to slavery must also have a voice because in our cultural collective they still survive.

An enslaved childhood

Every child born into slavery belonged to the mother—and to the slave owner. The maternal line was just as important as it had been in Roman times in relation to slaves. This was also the case in many African pre-colonial societies, including Egypt. Even though this fact of maternal "belonging" was there for every Africanist child born into slavery, they were not able to claim "mothering" as a right. Each child birthed on the plantation by right of law belonged to the slave owner. Most Africanist children did not realize this until around the age of eight or nine when they suddenly found themselves working in the fields or in the "big house." Up until this point life was relatively simple and could be physically comfortable.

The pleasures of early childhood and the equality of playmates which transcended color sometimes obscured the young slave's vision of bondage. During this period, many of the young blacks had no idea they were slaves. J. Vance Lewis wrote that on a Louisiana plantation during his early childhood:

> As a barefoot boy my stay upon the farm had been pleasant. I played among the wild flowers and wandered, in high glee, over hill and hollow, engaged with the beauty of nature, and knew not that I was a slave, and the son of a slave." ... Frederick Douglas said that during his childhood, "it was a long time before I knew myself to be a slave." This was true, he said, because "the first seven or eight years of the slave-boy's life are about as full of sweet content as those of the most favored and petted white children of the slaveholder."
>
> (Blassingame, 1972, p. 184)

This did not in any way prevent Africanist children from seeing the violence that occurred because physical and verbal abuse was a trademark of plantation life. Due to the randomness of the meting out of punishment, violent acts could be expected at any moment and could come from any number of sources. Former slave children reported that their own mothers had died because Africanist children had spoken about them in front of white children. These same white playmates, when speaking to their parents, had endangered the safety and lives of Africanist mothers, who could be whipped or killed for the "wrong words" spoken in secret against a white slave owner or his wife.

> As the children aged life began to change and they became more aware of their status. However, there were children such as Thomas Jones who had

never experienced the almost idyllic-like experience of some: "I was born a slave .... I was made to feel, in my boyhood's first experience, that I was inferior and degraded, and that I must pass through life in a dependent and suffering condition." ...

Those who were lucky enough to avoid Jones's experience in early childhood knew what he felt by the time they reached their teens. Many began working irregularly at light tasks before they were ten. After that age they usually started working in the fields. Since labor was the first, and irreparable, break in childhood equality in black–white relations.

(Blassingame, 1972, p. 185).

However, as previously stated the erratic display of violence on the plantation meant that the same kind of unpredictability existed for children. Most black children learned vicariously what slavery was long before this point. They were often terrified by the violent punishment meted out to the black men around them.

The beginning of Jermain Loguen's sense of insecurity and brutal awareness of what he was, for example, occurred when he saw a vicious white planter murder a slave and was cautioned to silence by his mother. The shock of seeing their parents flogged was an early reminder to many black children of what slavery was. When young William Wells Brown saw his mother flogged for being late going to the fields, he recalled that "the cold chills ran over me, and I wept aloud." The flogging Ball's mother received when he was four years old still retained its "painful vividness" to him forty-seven years later.

(Blassingame, 1972, p. 186)

There came a time in every slave child's life when he or she had to be "broken." This breaking, like training an animal to grow strong and then yield based on the trainer's wishes, would happen gradually and began at the age of ten years or sometimes sooner. In *Deep Like the Rivers: Education in the Slave Quarter Community, 1831–1865*, Thomas L. Webber says of this training:

Many planters did, however, begin the "breaking" process before the slave child was strong enough to do a full-hand's work. Most quarter children between the ages of six and ten were given miscellaneous chores around the plantation. They tended sheep, milk cows, gathered firewood, toted water, helped with the cooking, assisted at the nursery, swept the yard, ran errands, and generally did whatever little jobs were needed done from moment to moment.

(1978, p. 21)

From an early age black children were learning how to be efficient workers on the plantation. They were a young group of forced labor in training to further the financial success of the plantation owner. Due to this early training on the land and survival in terms of food and aspects of nature, the African men and women who survived acquired important skills for gaining their freedom from slavery. This became, over time, one of the main assets for becoming a runaway slave—one's ability to remain away from the plantation and take care of the physical body until finding safety in freedom.

Black children were taught how to survive by their mothers, as this was the most important factor of being a slave—this was survival in the hope of one day being free. This was part of African American cultural psychological experience since the early days of slavery. As generations bled into more generations of life spent on plantations and in slavery, the valued hope became one of freedom and in order to one day reach it, survival was essential. This type of survival required the defense of their parents and children were expressive of defending their parents or at least had such feelings.

> Listening to stories of runaways and seeing slaves interact in the quarters, the slave child had many models of behavior. In fact, he saw his parents playing two contradictory roles. In the quarters, for example, where he saw his parents most often, his father acted like a man, castigating whites for their mistreatment of him, being a leader, protector, and provider. On the few occasions when the child saw him at work the father was obedient and submissive to his master. Sometimes children internalized both the true personality traits and the contradictory behavioral patterns of their parents.
> Since, however, their parents' submission was on a shallow level of convenience directed toward avoiding pain, it was less important as a model of behavior than the personality traits they exhibited in the quarters.
> (Blassingame, 1972, p. 190)

Mother and child health

> Many slave mothers adhered to mores that made motherhood almost sacred, mores rooted in the black woman's African past. In tradition West Africa, mothers by virtue of their having and nurturing children, ensured the survival of the lineage, the consanguineal corporate group that controlled and dictated the use and inheritance of property, provided access to various political and/or religious offices, regulated marriages, and performed political and economic functions. Mothers were the genetically significant link between successive generations .... In all African societies having children meant having wealth, since their work translated into material gain.
> (White, 1998, p. 106)

African American slave children were usually brought into the world with the birthing help of older women slave midwives. This was a tradition in African society and continued in America. The African women who came to America as herbalists and healers had practiced traditional medicine for centuries before arriving in America. Within this tradition, women healers as part of the matriarchal overseeing women's health care, were always the first to be consulted about sick or pregnant women. Over time, concerned about those who they labeled "barren" women, slave owners began to consult medical doctors. Initially, these medical men were consulted about the physical needs of slaves who might be suffering from any number of illnesses, but they were not always the first point of call when a black man or woman was sick. In being called upon to treat illnesses and assist at births, Africanist women healers had philosophical beliefs that bound medicine/herbs to these beliefs.

Marie Jenkins Schwartz, in *Birthing a Slave*, writes:

> Slaves did not draw sharp distinctions between matters involving the body and the spirit, between physical and emotional well-being. Sickness might be viewed on the one hand as something gone wrong with bodily processes or on the other as the result of supernatural powers either deliberately or inadvertently inflicted.
>
> *(2009, p. 34)*

In the early 19th century medical doctors did not usually have any medical school training. Even those that did have training might not have any in the specialized area of midwifery. Many Americans grouped all medical and healer practitioners together. There were a range of services provided but the area of specialty pertaining to women's health—especially in the area of birthing—was controlled, if not overtly, by Africanist women healers. Schwartz says:

> When it came to women's health, the orthodox physician's biggest competitor was the midwife. In the South, most midwives were enslaved blacks with no formal training, especially in the country, where the majority of slaves lived …. By the 1840s obstetrics was receiving a separate emphasis. It had its own textbooks and had become part of the core curriculum of Southern medical schools, although often it was taught as a part of a general course on the diseases of women and children …. When it came to women's health, the knowledge of doctors entering practice was if anything more limited than other fields of study. Most had never witnessed a live birth or treat gynecological problems. Because elite women spurned inexperienced, the majority of medical men in all likelihood attended their first case or cases of childbirth in the slave quarter, thus *according black women an important role in the furthering of medical knowledge.*
>
> *(2009, pp. 36–37; emphasis added)*

Black women participated in the "furthering of medical knowledge" because responsibility for their care was shared between the doctor and the slave owner. The black woman patient had no ability to interject any of her wishes in the medical process or procedure for her own care. Medical doctors during the antebellum period were becoming wealthy due to their work on slave plantations. By joining in a relationship with the owners for the treatment of slaves they were becoming rich men who themselves envisioned become plantation owners. Though these men initially had limited experience and only a minimal amount of formal education regarding women's bodies, they gained experience working on the bodies of black women. As with all aspects of the plantation, the medical doctors who gradually began replacing traditional Africanist healers, became financially endowed due to their experimental work with black women. The medical knowledge that they acquired would almost never be applicable to black women because the best care once available due to experimentation on black women, was transferred to white women.

The care of enslaved Africanist women was possibly handled any number of ways. The interests of medical doctors in the 1840s added their presence to the plantation in addition to traditional healers as well as plantation owners. All three of these groups competed in differing ways to provide care to slaves. Owing to his desire for greater monetary rewards and status the doctor sought to become the primary health care practitioner for slaves. The plantation owner in hoping to reduce the intervention of the medical doctor and maintain power as the central figure of control on the plantation was not always so eager to have the medical doctor treat slave patients. However, the Africanist healer had the most sway with Africanist patients through centuries of providing care and healing:

> When medical conditions were not urgent or desperate, owners preferred to place their trust in the slave's root-and-herb doctor midwife, if only to save the expense of the physician's visit but also to save the trouble of imposing particular treatment that might meet resistance .... The fact that it was often difficult to obtain the services of a competent doctor encouraged the concept of self-sufficiency for both blacks and whites .... Particularly at the early onset of disease, during mild spells of illness, or in routine obstetric cases, owners left healing in the hands of slaves.
>
> (Schwartz, 2009, p. 51)

Over time, the interests of the slave owner turned more to increasing the number of children birthed on the plantation. There was still an interest in the overall care of slaves but female slaves acquired special significance because of the slave owners' plan for adding more slave children to his or her plantation. There were no moral codes that might inhibit this primarily financial interest on the part of the owner. He did believe he was providing care for *his* slaves and that the labor they provided him and that some of his economic wealth could be spent on ensuring their health. They were after all *his* producers of even more wealth. However, using enslaved healers successfully helped him to keep his expenses to a minimum. Furthermore, the medical doctor also had no moral code that prohibited his interest in increasing the plantation owner's "supply" of children.

The doctor could add wealth and status to his own medical practice by honing his ability to provide the slave owner with remedies for birthing more children and eliminating infertility. In joining together, the slave owner and medical doctor thus established their own immoral code of behavior that would affect the health care of generations of black women.

There were many ways for children to die on a plantation. Their rate of sickness was greater than that of white children. There was no intention to promote the death of black children as they were seen as adding to the profits of the plantation. However, they were vulnerable to much more physical harm on the plantation than others due to their age, exposure to the environment and potential physical abuse. The care of black children by their family and healer often reflected West African customs. In *The Myth of the Negro Past* Herskovits, quoting Puckett, states:

> In the Sea Islands and in Mississippi, according to one formant when a child is slow to walk you should bury him naked in the earth to his waist, first tying a string around his ankle. The same informants also speak of carrying a child to the doctor to have his tongue clipped when he is slow to talk. While sweeping is sometimes used beneficially one should never sweep the room while the child is asleep. The idea is that you will sweep him away, and this seems to be possibly a half-remembered notion of the African "dream-soul" which leaves the body during sleep. ...
>
> To "call" the soul of a child before going on a journey is routine in West Africa, and elaborate care must be taken on numerous other occasions to ensure that it stays with its owner and continue to exercise benevolence toward him .... Among the Yoruba, and in Dahomey, well-recognized rituals exist in which a person pays homage to his soul, while in the Gold Coast the patrilineal soul line is of equal importance with the matrilineal descent line.
>
> *(1958, p. 194)*

It is important to note the connection of soul and children. The rituals and recognition of spirituality that was brought by ancestors and left to American slave descendants continued to be alive in their collective cultural consciousness. In acknowledgement of the death of the physical body there remained a concurrent belief in the enjoined relationship of that which was spiritual and archetypal.

Archetypal grief

Mythology provides us with images of death as well as stories of heroism, creation myths and tales of different gods. Several of these images and stories are familiar to us. African myths generally originate from different countries across the continent and sometimes have a creation myth that ends in the bringing of death to human beings. Interestingly, this is oftentimes written as being the responsibility of a female. In *Mythology: An Illustrated Guide,*

> A woman is blamed for the arrival of death on Earth in a myth of the Dinka, cattle keepers of the southern Sudan. ...In the beginning, they say, the High

> God gave a grain of millet a day to a certain couple called Garang and Abuk, and this satisfied their needs. But Abuk greedily decided to plant more grain and in doing so accidently hit the High God with the end of her hoe. The deity was so angry that he withdrew to his present great distance humanity and sent a bluebird to sever the rope which at that time linked heaven and earth.
>
> (Willis, 1993, p. 269)

According to Egyptian folklore, Isis loses her son/lover in the Nile River that was created by her tears. The Mother of Sorrows is a Roman Catholic image of grief and mourning. This archetype represents the relationship of death and loss between the Virgin Mary and Jesus. The image of the Pieta by Michelangelo exemplifies at an aesthetic level the anguish of a mother who suffers the death of her child.

> Until recently, slave studies rarely discussed children's experiences in the trans-Atlantic slave trade. It has been estimated that one quarter of the slaves who crossed the Atlantic were children. Yet, a lack of sources and a perceived lack of importance kept their experiences in the shadows and left their voices unheard.
>
> (Colleen A. Vasconcellos, Item #141)

Even though the mythic stories and narratives may cast the shadow of guilt upon women for the loss and death of their own children, this goes against the reality of how most mothers love and care for their children. In the oppression of slavery, women collaborated to take care not only of their own children but also those of others within the Africanist plantation community who were related by blood or who had suffered the loss of their biological parent. It is important to attempt to correct historical "facts" when they are skewed. Frequently, these facts that have developed over the centuries are not the truth of the African or the African American women and parent.

There can be guilt feelings in the mother who loses her child even when she bears no responsibility for the death of her child. The reason for the death of children who died in captivity in Africa, during the Middle Passage and on the slave plantations had no connection with the parents of these children. Their deaths were caused by the historical incidence of an African Holocaust.

When I consider the grief experienced by the mothers who lost children in the African Holocaust, I think about their emotional bodies. The physical body is captured and the mind can be tortured by the trauma of the abusive captivity. This trauma includes a sense of helplessness, anger and fear.

The possibility of death for the mother as well as the loss of not just one child but *all* of her children would have pressed heavily on the heart of any enslaved mother. The nature of her grief in witnessing this possibility of the loss through death or sale of each child I believe would have been recreated over each generation. The presence of violence in each lifetime of *every* mother and child traveled with them, as did their emotional and biological selves. It would have been impossible to separate the intensity of trauma witnessed and/or experienced by enslaved Africanist people from their feelings. The emotions would have included fear, anxiety, guilt and shame. The constant witness bearing that the longevity of slavery required would also perhaps have numbed and disconnected them from the inner life that cried out for peace. I will not put myself aside in an objective space as I think about the possible emotional states of enslaved mothers and their children. This misalignment could only occur if I have not felt in my own life or in my work with Africanist patients the disassociation that stems from being worn down by racism experienced in the course of daily life. It is exhausting.

My life experience is overtly very different from my Southern ancestors. The ways in which it is similar happens mostly by way of a selective cultural consciousness and archetypal level that involves a felt sense of the relationship I have had with my parents and my ancestors. I was not born nor grew up in a vacuum separate from the history of my ancestors and my culture. My thoughts about this resonate with what Samuel Kimbles says in *Phantom Narratives: The Unseen Contributions of Culture to Psyche*:

> I introduce the concept of phantom narratives as a hybridized term expressing the background ambiguity of subject/objective, individual/group, politics/sociology, and personal biography and cultural history, conscious and unconscious, held together in an affective field. This affective field has a narrative structure with "deep and buried contents" (Chomsky, 1968) that operates at the level of the cultural unconscious and is structured by cultural complexes.
>
> *(2014, p. 17)*

As we now begin to be receptive to the idea of cultural complexes and allow our emotional selves to see the historical facts of the African Holocaust, we are present in an affective field which permits us to truthfully revisit—no matter how painful—what the phantoms of enslaved mothers and their children present to us. We must become believers of the truth of which our ancestors' stories speak. Historically, we have been taught not to trust our cultural phantom narratives. We have sometimes been made to believe that our traditions are mere "superstition" and without spiritual merit as we see others write about and develop theories—social and psychological—that incorporate indigenous philosophical beliefs.

The archetypal grief of enslaved mothers and their descendants are a part of our collective cultural suffering. This type of grief is nurtured and kept alive because of the conditions of the trauma which first began creating it through the pattern of a Mother of Sorrows archetype. The pattern has been in our human consciousness for a very long time—since the death of first child—Cain killing Abel; Mary holding Jesus at the foot of the cross; Isis clutching the dismembered parts of Horus in her hands. Mothers know how to love their children and they know how to grieve for their children. African American mothers have had centuries in which to embrace grief for the loss of their children. I believe that this type of grief, sustained for centuries within consciousness, makes it archetypal.

Judith A. Savage, in *Mourning Unlived Lives: A Psychological Study of Childbearing Loss*, addresses the emotional states of mothers whose children have died. She also looks at the archetypal dimension of such a loss. In reading her Jungian and sometimes Bowlby-related assessment account of the death of children, I worked to see the lines of connection between the archetypal, the sociological and the cultural of which she spoke. The context of my interest in this writing includes intergenerational cultural trauma and I was drawn to Savage's writing as Jungian.

The opening page of Savage's book contains a quote from Jung's *Memories, Dreams, Reflections*. I have included it here because I think that it goes the heart of contemplating the death of children and mourning:

> A categorical question is being put to (humankind), and (we are) under no obligation to answer it. To this end (we) ought to have a myth about death, for reason shows (us) nothing but the dark pit into which (we are) descending. Myth, however, can conjure up other images for (us), helpful and enriching pictures of life in the land of the dead. If we believe in them, or greet them with some measure of credence, we are being just as right or just as wrong as someone who does not believe in them. But while the one who despairs marches toward nothingness, the one who has placed .... faith in the archetype follows the tracts of life and lives right into one's own death. Both, to be sure, remain in uncertainty, but the one lives against one's instincts, the other with them.
>
> *(1989, p. v)*

Savage continues:

> It is common experience, at least for a time, the ongoing presence of the deceased. Thus depending on the cultural attitude toward such an experience, that is whether the presence of such spirits is collectively regarded as beneficial or detriment most cultures provide for a social sanction of these phenomena, and appropriate behavior in relation to them is prescribed.
>
> *(Ibid., p. 45)*

Meanwhile, Savage maintains that Neumann's *archetype of the way* is significant as a central metaphor of mourning and a "paradigm for mourning." This archetype represents the "dangerous darkness" of what Savage calls "primitive rituals," the goddess enactment of mourning, followed by *search, recovery and rebirth*. As an aspect of the *archetype of the way*, "Like ancient man's initiation mysteries, grief also seeks to understand and experience the healing, transformative nature of the numinous" (ibid., p. 47; emphasis in the original). In her discussion of the archetypal patterns of mourning, Savage states that there are three phases which include the initial phase of loss of the child, "Searching," which can also be described as "Yearning" or "Longing." These stages are described thus:

The mourner's open expression of sadness is collectively tolerated. Lasting a few days or weeks, the denial mechanisms eventually loosen and the mourner begins to accept the reality of the loss. Together, these varied and intense early emotional reactions to the loss combine to create, as in the first phase of any initial ritual, a period of disorganization or disorientation within the conscious personality. The following stage, that of Searching, also known as Yearning or Longing, is more enduring is particularly distressful to parents, especially mothers, who have lost children. Phenomenologically, this period is experienced as an unyielding ache in the mother's empty arms, or an intense heartache as symbolized by the Seven Swords presaged by Simeon that would pierce the heart of Mary, the Mother of Jesus, following his crucifixion. The behaviors of mourning that are constellated by the archetype of the Search include wandering, cutting of hair, dressing in black, being "unkempt," and relentlessly weeping. Its affects include depression, crying, anger, confusion, and pain.

(Ibid., pp. 49–50)

One of the features of child loss may be the reoccurring thought that you as a parent could have prevented this loss. Savage says that this is especially true and "the child's death remains experienced, on some level, as a failure of their parental protection" (ibid., p. 53). I imagine that this sense of failure accompanied by guilt would have become a presence in mothering slaves who lost their children through no fault of their own but who also felt responsible for their lives because they had birthed them into the world. How much of a part would reason have played in mediating a sense of guilt over the death of the children lost to parents in slavery? I wish I could know with certainty concerning the feeling of guilt by these mothers.

Parents being described by Savage were not enslaved nor experienced cultural trauma. They had experienced the death of their children but not for centuries. This is a premise of archetypal grief. It becomes embodied because it is intergenerational and it is cultural. We have very few records of African American dreams that provide a Searching theme as Savage has recorded in her book. She did, however, say that she had found that dreams of searching for the dead child and related dreams were "common" among women who had lost their children due to death. Would this have been true for mothering slaves? I cannot say. Perhaps historical dream research studies of African Americans will provide us with some answers to this question.

One of the differences between children lost to parents in contemporary times and those lost during slavery are the children sold away from their mothers. This was always a threat to mothering slaves—the sale of their children. For all the stories which address the occurrence of enslaved families remaining together, history has shown us that the selling off of children away from families was entirely up to the slaver. How are we to define and understand the emotional anguish of these slave mothers? In considering the archetypal pattern of Searching, where does the archetypal grief over children who had been sold find a place?

In her description of the mother's level of self-care during this period of grieving, Savage mentions the physical appearance of the mother as unkempt. Since this is related to the body, feelings of the body emerge in imagery according to Savage.

> It is common for parents who have lost a child at birth, produced a deformed or handicapped child, miscarried, or remained infertile, to unconsciously experience their bodies as *defectus incubus* (defective incubator), which then causes to remain unwilling to have other children or, if they do, to live in dreadful fear of the outcome.
>
> *(1989, p. 61; italic in the original)*

Under the conditions of slavery, we can read how mothering slaves were reluctant to have more children and sometimes wished death on the ones they had brought into the world. Is this then a part of the intergenerational archetypal grief pattern as regards black women and their relationship towards their bodies?

The story narratives of mothering slaves seldom offer a telling of their emotional states. Even if this was done, this aspect of the narrative—the omission of mother's feelings and emotions— did not appear to the narrator to be of much consequence; therefore, as readers we are usually left without the emotional expression of the mothers who lost their children through death or sale.

Rage as a part of any grief is typical, Savage noted that this is especially true in the case of mothers who have lost their children as a result of murder. In a study of childhood death Savage references a study by Knapp who carried out research with parents of murdered children. His findings of this include several factors which make the emotion of rage so dominant in the circumstance of murdered children: the suddenness of the loss; violence; intentionality of the murder; absence of choice; and the helplessness of the victim (Knapp, 1986). I would say that all of these factors are intertwined with many of the deaths of African and African American children—those on the Middle Passage crossings and those who survived the voyage only to face death on the plantation. What of the rage of these mothering slaves? Would this not be a part of *their* grief?

"Crying is such an essential aspect of grief that mourning cannot be imagined without it. Therefore, the absence of crying is generally considered a strong indication of a psychological disturbance" (Savage, 1989, p. 64). We cannot know (yet) from the history of mothering slaves how many cried their grief. There are few records.

Maybe like with all other aspects of mothering slaves, their emotional lives proved unimportant to historical recorders writing down their narratives. Perhaps there are few who have completed the research in this area of women's studies and more research is needed. In looking at Savage's archetypal pattern of Searching as a part of grief I wonder about the cases of aborted grief that mothering slaves must have experienced. This unnatural stopping of such a natural process as the death or sale of one's child(ren), must have been extraordinary. We know from slave narratives that care given to birthing women was inconsistent and we also know that their primary function following birthing—whether the child was dead or alive—was returning to work as slave labor for the plantation. How often did these mothers who had just given birth, bury their emotional suffering deep within selves and return to working the fields? Where was the place for their solace and their grief?

There are stories about enslaved women who returned to the fields following the live birth of their children. What of the mothers who lost their children to auctions and death—where are their stories of grief?

The experience of Africanist people shaped by the trauma of a holocaust and the deaths of many children opens up a line of questions that can only lead us to deeper and more intensive self-exploration. As we think about the archetype and try to find a comparable personal experience of individual or collective trauma, what happens? What is the energy that we can identify? How does the pattern of such a trauma show itself in our lives? This is particularly relevant given that the death witnessed by African Americans was genocidal.

I do believe that for those within an Africanist cultural complex, there is an acceptance of myths about death. This myth accepts that death is part of life. Whether this acceptance comes from the African myths told long before the arrival of slaves on American soil or which live only through the story's changing and retelling in slave cabins, there exists an unbroken flow of a connection with death that speaks to continuity. In the Beng tradition, children and those recently dead, live together in a compatibility that addresses co-existence in death and life. I think this is a myth that honors both aspects of human consciousness. The cultural trauma of the African Holocaust created within the Africanist psyche a further deepening of belief as regards the afterlife, as well as the before life. In a Nigerian mythology of creation, we know who we are before birth and we must through our spiritual work in our human bodies seek to remember what our soul has been sent to earth to experience and help us create as humans.

In the Africanist cultural complex there is a place for understanding the shortness of life and a respect for death. I believe that this too comes from the centuries of having to balance living with dying in such a deeply personal manner. In slave narratives we can see how death was a very frequent circumstance in plantation life. The oral recordings of former slaves are full of the images and words taken into consciousness from being witnesses to the torture and murder they had seen. Death was very familiar in their plantation lives—this was true for both adults and children. In these narratives, there is usually an absence of the emotional trauma experienced at witnessing someone's death.

The story of the telling of exact facts appears to remain the only thing worth telling. It is possible that this is due to a dissociation from having seen so much violence and death and/or an understanding that in the round of life and death, there was another place on the other side of the life of slavery that was much better—the afterlife promised hope as part of life's continuum.

9

MOTHER, DAUGHTER, SON

> Oh ye not, oh, my favored sisters,
> Just a plea, a prayer or a tear,
> For mothers who dwell 'neath the shadows
> Of agony, hatred and fear?
> *Frances E. W. Harper (1825–1911)*

Mother

In "Aspects of the Feminine," Jung says,

> Mother is mother-love, *my* experience and *my* secret. Why risk saying too much, too much that is false and inadequate and beside the point, about that human being who was our mother, the accidental carrier of that great experience which includes herself and myself and all mankind, and indeed the whole of created nature, the experience of life whose children we are?
> *(CW9i, para. 172; emphasis in the original)*

Our mothers are our secrets while still belonging to the generations of mothers who have come before them and who will follow. It is being proven with more and deeper scholarly research that the First Mother was a black mother. I do believe that when we can change some unknown instance into a more reasonable point of information, then we can change consciousness. One of the most destructive aspects of racism and our inability to see and continue to work with our racial complexes is denial of that which is obvious. If our human race initially appeared on the African continent it only follows that our First Parents originated there and were black. When we attempt to disavow rational information like this, refusing to accept the inevitability of such progressive clear facts, then we remain stuck in complexes which keep us psychological prisoners.

Those who might accept the First Mother as black worked laboriously to make Her, through placement of her lineage only through Greek mythology, not *really* black. In the history of Egypt, not only were the Nubians rarely acknowledged by white scholars as the first people of Egypt, but history was reconstructed so that the Egyptians became the *recipients* of Greek mythology and cultural influences. Slowly the wheel of history is turning to reveal that the opposite is in fact the truth. In *The Destruction of Black Civilization: Great Issues of a Race from 4500 B.C. to 2000 A.D.*, Chancellor Williams discusses the geographical and social movements within early Ethiopia and Egypt:

> Egypt, as pointed out before, was the North-eastern region of ancient Ethiopia. The six cataracts of the Nile were the great watermarks in the heartland of the Blacks from whence African culture spread over the continent, but nowhere was it pronounced as in Egypt. This northern sector of the Ethiopian empire had been the object of world attention from the earliest times. The fact was that it was in the center of the crossroads from all directions leading into Africa from Asia and Europe. The great agricultural system that was developed along the overflowing Nile was one of the sources of the wealth to support the great cultural advances. The other was the gold mines below the First Cataract. This was also the magnet that drew Caucasian peoples from many lands. As these increased in number and variety, the undermining of black power was accelerated …. The melting of the races began around the northern perimeter. The end result was always the same: The Blacks were pushed to the bottom of the social, economic and political ladder whenever and wherever the Asians and their mulatto off springs gained control. Scheme of weakening the Blacks by turning their half-white brother against them cannot be overemphasized because it began in the early times and it became the universal practice of whites, and it still one of the cornerstones in the edifice of white power. The white Asians were generally very proud of their sons by black women. But these black mothers remained slaves, while their mulatto sons and daughters were born and, moreover classified as "white." As such, they formed a social class that, while never recognized as equal with the "real whites," had just about all the other privileges of free men.
>
> *(1987, pp. 59–61)*

I have included a detailed extract from the abovementioned work by Williams because it is rare or perhaps almost impossible to obtain through casual sources an understanding of how the cultures of Africa were formed. This formation developed in an intentional manner that was influenced by ethnicity, even as far back as 4,000 BC. It is only with facts of how Africa really began millenniums ago are we able to find a place of understanding in the 21st century. We are unlikely to find out much about the mythologies of Africa or its people from the "shortened" version of American history that we learn in our primary and secondary schools. I believe a part of this is the focus on not providing an accurate history of African civilization because of the African Holocaust of slavery. The disruption to the American collective psyche and the African diaspora shows itself in our racial relationships and collective anguish regarding racism. In order to begin to understand how we continue to find ourselves in this situation requires a knowledge that goes beyond American history. It will teach us very little about Africanist cultural complexes or collective. It is not a diversion to walk down the historical path of ancient African history. On this path we will see social patterns that we thought were "new" and yet find that they have existed for thousands of years. In our understanding of archetypes and mythology and their presence in human consciousness, we must also accept that the narratives of early life reflected the unconscious. Mythologies and legends grew out of the stories of a people who carried, changed and influenced them in the telling of these stories.

> When the genius of Kemetic Egyptian civilization was rediscovered by Europe in the 18th and 19th centuries, this threatened return of the repressed was handled differently. Egypt was mentally and "scientifically" taken out of Africa and made an extension of European and Middle Eastern history and development. It became "Egypt *and* Africa."
>
> Along with this came a sudden interest in Indian culture and the Sanskrit language. The Indo-Aryan connection to India was heightened, and slowly a Caucasian genesis was seen in Hindu civilization. The Indigenous African was erased from the teaching of history and the unfoldment of human civilization. This subtle psychological process continues to this day on a large scale. With a few notable exceptions, in the Eurocentric tradition, it was simply inconceivable that a highly evolved civilization that gave light to the mind could have its genesis in a dark and mysterious world and then move in an African migration down toward the Mediterranean. This is despite the fact that the Romans did not come until Caesar, around 30 B.C.E., that the Greeks did not come in mass numbers before Alexander in 333 B.C.E., that the Jews did not come to be known before Abraham and Joseph .... By that time the Kemetic lens of the human mind had already developed several written scripts, astronomy, medicine, mathematics, mummification, a form of biological psychiatry, a precise calendar, the pyramids, and by the 8th century B.C.E. in the 25th Dynasty, had made contact with peoples from southern India to the Americas. Such awareness must be repressed if you are to hold people in bondage and justify the belief that they are an inferior race.
>
> *(Bynum, 2012, p. 80)*

The archetypes themselves reflected the developing consciousness of the people and their experiences of human life. Their cultures presented the archetypal forms and patterns of the deepest consciousness in service of furthering how we might join and live with one another from within ourselves and without in our community collective.

The archetypal event of American slavery ruptured both the in-dwelling development of the Africanist individual as well as the cultural group. As we continue to seek answers to philosophical questions created by the mere fact of our human existence—even without cultural trauma—it is essential to know our past because it presently influences our individual as well as group development. This is especially true for the group cohesiveness that belongs to mothers as a group with its own rite of passage, rituals and *inner eye* of perception.

In *The Motherline*, Naomi Ruth Lowinsky addresses the influence of belonging to the motherline and raises important questions:

> What does it mean for modern women to speak in the mother tongue, to honor the richness of the Motherline, to hear the voices of the lost women in our souls? It means to sink down into a world outside ordinary time, to sink into what we feel in our bodies and in our emotions, to allow ourselves to see with the inner eye as well as the outer, to delve down into the forbidden areas of our experience, to attend to those things that make us ashamed.
>
> *(1992, p. 38)*

As women we are always faced with these kinds of questions. This is true even of women who are not birth mothers. The recognition of an ancestral mother, many ancestral mothers, can be a powerful energy field from which *to hear the voices of the lost women in our souls*. What do their voices wish to say—do they want to express their historical, archetypal experiences? What is it that we need at this point in our century to help us to meet the challenges of being women in a society which is becoming more misogynistic as the years pass by? Questions by Lowinsky support the asking of more questions that can focus our attention on motherhood and the matriarchal line. Not only the easy questions but also those which are difficult, and are related to mothering slaves.

> It is possible that the religious ideas of ancient Crete and Egypt originated in black Africa. During 7000 to 6000 BC, the Sahara was a rich and fertile land, and a great civilization flourished there. Images of the Horned Goddess (who became Isis of Egypt) have been found in caves on a now-inaccessible plateau in the center of what is now the Sahara desert. When the earlier fertile land dried out, probably as a result of climatic change, the people spread out from this center, and wherever they settled they brought with them the religion of the Black Goddess, the Great Mother of Africa.
>
> *(Sjoo and Mor, 1987, p. 21)*

Though all of our matriarchal lines originate from the same ancient black Mother and our goddess mythologies do sometimes overlap, we can be separated by time and culture. As I read the mythologies of African goddesses of the Yoruba tradition, I seek to find a connection, the place where we bond through the archetypal energy of culture.

What is evoked through my experiences due not only to the archetype of slavery but also to childbirth and the subsequent life that is based on my and my sisterhood's archetypal energy within our cultural complex? We have begun to explore these and similar questions in the last few decades, thinking on how these questions might have some significance in our psychic lives and are thus related to our humanness.

The archetypal mother is she who carries us from one generation to the next passing along the attributes of nurture and protection. In the face of the African Holocaust, this mother archetype was influenced by the archetype of slavery. The results of the activation of group cultural racial complexes caused an African population catastrophe. When the African Holocaust was first spoken of in these terms there was reaction against the suggestion that it was as horrific as this. The time that had elapsed since the African Middle Passage made some writers and others engaged in open social discussion want to forget this holocaust. The desire to forget and minimally recall slavery was defended by those who did not wish to give any historical credence to the cultural trauma caused by the African Holocaust. This too is changing. As African and African American writers become more productively focused as historical writers it is possible to create works—whether sculpture or teaching that identify the accurate results of slavery and its aftermath.

It becomes possible to speak more openly and without being "shouted down" about an African history that included black Egypt, and medical and scientific accomplishments as well as intellectually enlightened achievements that have their origins in black Africa.

The mythology of the African goddesses—the archetypal mother—offers women an opportunity to learn more about themselves. The history of consciousness regarding women mythology—including black women—continues to be written. The archetypal grief of black women carried through generations *can* be influenced by the archetypes. If the interruption of societies in African can occur through the archetypal energy of slavery and its racial complexes, then it can interrupt a false narrative regarding black women. This shift in consciousness would see more of the images of black women descending from the line of goddesses and queens, from the African Great Mother rather than the jezebel or mammy.

> Throughout Europe—especially Eastern Europe, but also in Spain, France and Italy—we can find Black Madonnas. People have local legends to explain the blackness of these Virgin Mary statues, including the ingenious ideas that the icon is charred, the miraculous survivor of a terrible fire. Jungian interpreters would see the blackness as a "subconscious" reference to the dark side of something or other—the moon, no doubt. It is rarely speculated that a real, historic blackness of the early goddesses of Egypt and Africa is being recalled …. these Black Madonnas …. are solid iconic remains of the ancient time

when the religion of the Black Goddess ruled Africa and from thence, much of the rest of the world.

(Sjoo and Mor, 1987, pp. 31–32)

Daughter

In many African societies we can still note the initiation rituals of young girls that introduced them into their communities in preparation for becoming wives and mothers. One of the African traditions that initially survived the American slave experience was initiation puberty rites and rituals for girls and boys. With the passage of time the rituals associated with the initiation into adulthood became less possible even though the mothering slaves who remembered the rituals that had been passed down from one generation to the next, probably still desired their use as meaningful life markers. The reality of slavery intervened and affected culturally established coming of age rituals. Deborah Gray White, in her chapter entitled "The Life Cycle of the Female Slave," states:

> The memories of these former slaves suggest that girls were not kept close to home in the exclusive company of women and were not socialized at an early age to assume culturally defined feminine roles. Black girls on the plantation spent most of their time in a sexually integrated atmosphere .... This easy integration of boys and girls is perhaps understandable in the context of their future plantation roles. Since both girls and boys were expected to become field hands, and they often found themselves doing similar work in later life, it is not surprising that as children they did the same chores and played the same games .... This does not mean that parents did not relate to girls and boys differently—there is no way of knowing if they did nor did not. It does seem, however, that parents were more concerned that children, regardless of sex, learned to walk the tightrope between the demands of the whites and expectations of the blacks without falling too far in either direction. It was probably more important for nine-year-old girls to learn that conversations among blacks in the slave quarters were not for white consumption, than for them to learn that cooking was a "feminine" activity.
>
> *(1998, p. 93)*

Perhaps the archetypal grief of enslaved mothers was the loss of initiation rites through which girls made the transition into womanhood. I imagine that the feminine emptiness created by such a loss might possibly add to cycles of psychological emotional suffering that remaining nameless would be present in the African American psyche.

In *The Dreams of African American Women: Heuristic Study in Dream Imagery*, the chapter entitled "Reframing African Mythology" discusses African mythology and its connection with initiation rites:

An African community that appears to have a regenerative spirit was discussed in Kevin Maxwell's *Bemba Myth and Ritual: The Impact of Literacy on an Oral Culture* (1983). Maxwell traced the development of oral traditions controlled by Africans to written language controlled by missionaries and colonial administrators. In an oral-aural culture such as Bemba, where so much emphasis is placed on sound, there is equal emphasis on sound-producing activities such as drumming, singing and storytelling.

In the Bemba creation myth, black and white races initially live together, but the whites eventually leave. Mumbi Mukasa falls from the sky and marries, producing three sons and one daughter. In his analysis of this myth, Maxwell (1983) states that the myth describes the "origins of the basic features of Bemba culture." It contains tribal geography, genealogy, and central African "mythological clichés such as incest, white magic, seeds in the hair." Through their religion, members of the society express respect for the hierarchy of its crocodile clan, observe sacred territory, and re-enact "archetypal" values of the ancestors through ritual. Mumbi Mukasa, the mythological hero, joins earth and heaven and lives comfortably with animals—both the elephant (land+water) and the crocodile (land+water). He creates marriage, sex and procreation, establishing the divinity of the matrilineage.

Maxwell (1983), in his analysis of Bemba mythology, referenced the theories of Luc De Heusch. The towers' collapse is a sign of dysfunction between heaven and Earth—cosmic discontinuity. In the myth, East is cosmological and analogous to heaven, to which the Divine withdraws. Maxwell stated that the journey motif of the myth is "authentically Bemba" and that the myth discloses the destructive consequences of adultery. In this regard, it is possible to observe clearly the influence of Levi-Strauss in Maxwell's analysis of Bemba myths.

Maxwell (1983) saw a connection between ritual and myth. Both are narratives that develop an elaborate symbolic system. He quoted Eliade in stating his own position regarding ritual, which Eliade identified as the "dramatic re-enactment of myth." Symbols carry tradition and authority. Each ritual defines some element of the creation myth and in this way continuously reinforces the power of cultural or mythological symbology. Maxwell noted that there are hermeneutical differences between written description of myths and rites and their performances. In a detailed description of a female puberty rite, *cisungu*, the mythic comes alive through ritual.

The first element of the *cisungu* ritual is one of transformation. A specific pattern of time suggests preliminal separation, liminal transition, and postliminal reincorporation, all as a part of the transformation taking place during the rite. Themes of the ritual itself include sacredness of female sexuality, centrality of matrilineal descent, honoring the traditional duty of wife and mother, and veneration of the spirits. Maxwell (1983) explored the symbols of the rite, noting that the sun signifies immortality, as does the snake. The rites of the young women directly connect with the actions of Mukulumpe—at the sign of their first menstruation, the women run into the forest and, as Mukulumpe imprisoned his daughter, so too are the initiates locked in huts. In describing the oral features of *cisungu*, Maxwell identified *mbusa*, sacred pots and the sacred emblems that are hand-painted on the pots. Each initiate has a specific poem and dance that the initiate is given to memorize and recite at selected times. The tradition of honoring the elder is shown when senior women from the community take an active leadership role in the initiation rites of the young women. The word *mbusa* itself means "things handed down." During the ceremony, the sacred pots are handed down from seniors to initiates, who receive them on their heads. Each pot is decorated with seeds representing wisdom. In the ritual, the initiates' mothers sow seeds in the garden, and the girls lie down and place their heads against the seeded mounds.

In the final section, Maxwell offered his own thoughts and ideas regarding these rituals from his personal observations and implementation of the guidelines established by Levi-Strauss and earlier mythologists. According to Maxwell's research, literacy has not displaced the dominance of the oral tradition. The strength and longevity of mythology combined with religion has created a powerful force in community life surpassing the effects of written language.

Brewster (2011)

Initiation rituals changed with the advance of slavery. However, it has been noted that African cultural customs were able to survive in certain parts of South America and Brazil and the West Indies whereas in America this was not the same circumstance.

In the chapter entitled "The Acculturative Process" in *The Myth of the Negro Past*, Herskovits discusses the difference between customs that were retained and those that failed to continue in some form in parts of North America:

> What caused the differences between the several parts of the New World in retention of African custom? Though the answer can only be sketched …. the effective factors are discernible. They are four in number: climate and topography; the organization and operation of the plantations; the numerical ratios of Negroes to whites; and the extent to which the contacts between Negroes and white since a given area took place in a rural or urban setting.
>
> (1958, p. 111)

I believe that the custom of initiation puberty rites were particularly affected by the "organization and operation of the plantation," through the concerted effort to erase what Herskovits called "Africanisms" in the very early days of slavery. The intense effort to remove all signs of African culture inadvertently included initiation rituals. Given their treatment of African and African American women I do not believe that traders or slavers had any knowledge of African rituals or, if this knowledge was present, any respect for rites of passage and their accompanying rituals. Black humanity was already invisible by the time of the early capturing of

Africans into slavery for delivery to America's shores. Whatever cultural attributes of Africans were present in the psyche of Africans began an "initiation" of a different and more painful kind at enslavement. The ability to practice one's religion and other customs were now forbidden and severely restricted.

The work of *remembering* is crucial to African American women attempting to make our past not only honorable but also elevated. The reality of the treatment of African people arriving and later living in America was purely dishonorable. The reverse occurred where Africans were made to believe that they should be lowered beneath whites partly due to their social customs. A necessary aspect to remembering is locating places that still do have African culture intact and using these survivals to remember our early African diaspora ancestors who due to the trauma of slavery were able to focus only on survival and freedom. In the struggle to maintain life under slavery—especially with the sexual assault of Africanist women—the possibility of saving the rite of passage of puberty would be impossible. Because of the nature of cruelty in American slavery in regards to black women's bodies, almost all African customs would be rooted out in service to the economic needs of the plantation. Young girls were no more permitted to have any rights to their own bodies than older women. Even if the rite of passage of puberty and its rituals could have been remembered, it would have been very difficult for African American females to honor these rituals due to the very nature of slavery towards black women. Fertility and all connected "rights" of childbirth were in the final determination under the control of white owners and doctors:

> Mary was greatly agitated in 1822 upon the onset of labor; the midwife attending her could not control her violent flailing. Her agitation ceased about 11 p.m., but so did her contractions. She continued to moan and to complain of a steady pain throughout the night, however, and vomited occasionally. Twenty-six hours after the labor pains had begun and fifteen hours following the cessation of contractions, a physician arrived to take charge. Concluding that Mary had been injured by her flailing, John Overton, M.D., of Nashville, decided not to wait any longer for "nature to furnish any assistance." The accoucheur turned the infant who came into the world feet first. Soon the patient started to hemorrhage. Once again the doctor intervened, this time to stop the flow. Three days later the doctor returned to treat Mary for what he described as a tumor—most likely resulting from the accumulation of fluids. The enslaved patient was eighteen years old. She survived, but she never became pregnant again, although according to Overton she menstruated following the incident. The doctor published the story nineteen years after the events in the *Western Journal of Medicine and Surgery*.
>
> (Schwarz, 2009, p. 143)

The most obvious component that appears to be missing from stories of mothering slaves are their emotional selves. It is as if the grief, tears and sorrow of these women must also be "scrubbed" clean as Herskovits says was attempted with

African culture. The descriptions of black women's lives under the persecution of slavery usually fail to relay to the reader the emotional impact of slavery on family, culture and their very own bodies. I think that is why it is important to bring the deep loss of enslaved mothers, children and descendants more into the light, out of shadow, through attention to archetypal grief. In the quotation above, there is no mention of Mary's psychological or emotional state—just that she survived *and* had no more children. This is the obvious surface narrative of Mary—what of her emotional body and psychic wellness? If we continue to read the stories about slavery and our ancestors without addressing their emotional and archetypal selves regarding the impact of slavery, how will we ever be able to focus our attention on what haunts us in the 21st century? The attempt to maintain a societal amnesia does not serve us as a cultural collective. Our work is to remember. Even as others may say that we do not have an African culture to reference, even as we hear that we are savages—still, even as we must struggle to bring our hidden past out of the shadow and into the light, we must seek to engage in remembering and voicing this remembrance in any way that we can. The archetypal grief of mothering slaves is real and I believe it is passed on down the generations as a part of our cultural trauma. This cannot be washed away.

Son

As I write about girls and women in this book, I think about the male children who entered, survived or died in slavery. I also think about the enslaved boys who grew into men and were our ancestors. What of these boys? In the same way that enslaved girls were initially raised on the plantations, so too were the sons of mothering slaves. In the early years of life, as previously noted, enslaved boys and girls played together with white children on the plantation. It wasn't until black children became older that they were separated by ethnicity and therefore by division of labor. Lunsford Lane, a former slave, says in *Deep Like the Rivers*:

> On the 30th of May, 1803, I was ushered into the world; but I did not begin to see the rising of its dark clouds, nor fancy how they might be broken and dispersed until some time afterwards. My infancy was spent upon the floor, in a rough cradle, or sometimes in my mother's arms. My early boyhood in playing with other boys and girls, colored and white, in the yard, and occasionally doing such little matters of labor as one of so young years could. I knew no difference between myself and the white children; nor did they seem to know any in turn.
>
> *(Webber, 1978, pp. 19–20)*

Many former slaves related similar stories about their childhood. The main similarity was that during the early years, race was a unimportant factor in that black and white children were allowed to play together. One former slave spoke of the intentionality of this situation.

> Despite these "darker clouds" which overcast the early childhood years, few slave children seem to have realized the full significance of their slave status until their slave training begin in earnest. On many large plantations those children destined to become fieldhands were left to grow strong and healthy until between the ages of ten and fourteen.
>
> (Ibid., p. 21)

It appears to have been a consistent pattern that many enslaved children, with the exception of future "house" slaves, were encouraged to engage in play with minimum work tasks until they reached at least eight years of age—some even ten. Most, including Frederick Douglass, spoke of the shock at making the transition from a play-filled childhood without the labor-intensive life of adult slaves around them to suddenly finding themselves full-time working slaves.

As they grew older and stronger, children working in the fields would be given regular but smaller tasks than those carried out by adults. Webber observed that all fieldhands "are divided into four classes, according to their physical capacities. The children beginning as 'quarter-hands,' advancing to 'half-hands,' and then to 'three-quarter-hands,'; and finally, when mature, and abled-bodied, healthy and strong, to 'full-hands'" (1978, p. 23).

The systematic use of both boy and girl children did become more obvious as they grew older and this had a good deal to do with gender in terms of sexual relations. Many reports of early childhood relations say that pre-puberty boys and girls most often slept as well as played together. As they began to approach puberty, this changed. Young girls and boys began to be encouraged to become sexual partners. The support of the slave-owner-promoted eventuality was seen by mothering slaves as something they wished to forego for as long as possible. It has been noted that young African girls and early Africanist females developed a later menstruation cycle and so this made engaging in sexual relations with a resulting pregnancy less likely. However, this did not decrease the possibility of sexual assault on black female children.

Boy children had loving relationships with their mothers as did girls. Perhaps the fear of forced future sexual behaviors made mothers less concerned for their boy children in this way and more anxious for their physical well-being in terms of being beaten, tortured and/or murdered. This is of course not to say that this might not happen to females. The care with which enslaved mothers had to provide their children was all around and included their feeding, clothing, protection from outside abuse and education about life. The desire for freedom from slavery was an influence on the way in which mothers taught their children and what they taught them. In considering both slavery and freedom as archetypes, it seems a possible factor that these archetypal energies would seek to create a psychic balance in the internal struggle of one against the other. This would have happened internally as well as in the outside world. Male children who grew up with a close, protective connection with their mothers were oftentimes taught to seek freedom for themselves but these children did not wish to leave their mothers in slavery.

Slave mothers, were, of course, held in even greater esteem by their children. Frequently, small children fought overseers who were flogging their mothers. Even when they had an opportunity to escape from bondage, many slaves refuse to leave their mothers. As a young slave, William Wells Brown did not run away because he "could not bear the idea" of leaving his mother. He felt that "after she had undergone and suffered so much for me would be proving recreant to the duty which I owed to her" (Blassingame, 1972, p. 191).

One former slave, Jacob Stroyer, tells how his father spoke of freedom as coming in the future "though he may not live to see it" (Blassingame, 1972, p. 190) Stroyer said that he was encouraged not to fight back by his father against their plantation owner but rather to pray and hope for freedom. According to Stroyer, his "heart swelled with the hope of the future, which made every moment seem an hour to me" (ibid.).

African American enslaved sons and fathers came from an African ancestral lineage that included initiation rites. These rites had a basic underpinning of philosophy and spiritual beliefs that prepared them to move emotionally within from children to adults and socially to enter into communities as responsible adults. The rite of passage of male children included rituals that generally through a number of African societies included circumcision. In *African Religions and Philosophy*, John S. Mbiti discusses the initiation rites of passage of children from different African communities including Akamba (Kamba), Maasai and Ndebele. In his chapter on initiaton and puberty rites, Mbiti provides the reason for the rites. I believe it is important to note the emotional and behavioral lives of ancestors because their need for ritual is also our 21st-century need for ritual. When we can remember something of these rituals, we can perhaps find more meaning in daily life. We can perhaps understand our own possession of something archetypal that takes hold of us as we work at transforming our deeper selves—not only fulfilling egoic wishes. Mbiti says, "Initiation rites have many symbolic meanings, in addition to the physical drama and impact" (1989, p. 118). These meanings introduce and reinforce community life, knowledge of religious beliefs and a sense of responsibility to the family and community. In addition, the rites prepare children for entering into life as married individuals who will become parents.

In the Akamba tradition, the initiation rites involve three stages and the first takes place when children are between four and seven years of age. According to Mbiti, after circumcision, "public rejoicing" takes place which includes "making libation and food offerings to the living-dead." The cutting of the foreskin of boys is a symbol of the leave-taking of childhood. (1989, p. 119) The pain of the circumcision, the blood and connection with the cutting of the umbilical cord all are to remind the boy/son that he must be strong as he becomes a man who will one day have his own children. Through his blood he has contact with the living-dead and this will continue through his lifetime. The second initiation will happen at a later date that varies. Mbiti says this second initiation is mostly educational and the boy lives away from the village for several days. Teachers provide what is known as "brooding over the initiates," and in teaching how to deal with fear, the boy face a monster—the "mbusya" (rhinoceros).

> On the second day [of initiation], they have to face a frightening monster known as "mbusya." In some parts of the country only the boys go through this experience, while in other parts both boys and girls do. This is a man-made structure of sticks and trees, from the inside of which someone makes fearful bellows like those of a big monster. The initiates do not know exactly what it is, for this is one of the secrets of the ceremony.
>
> *(Ibid., p. 121)*

Other activities include hunting and learning through symbolic sexual play about male-female sexuality. A final ritual during this time occurs at the sacred tree:

> The rite of the sacred tree is a reminder of the religious life, and a symbolic visit to the living-dead and the spirits who are thought to live there .... The slight cut on the sex organs at the sacred tree indicates the sacredness of sex, in the sight of God, the spirits, the living-dead and the humanity community. The return home is like an experience of resurrection: death is over, their seclusion is ended, and now they rejoin their community as new men and women, fully accepted and respected as such.
>
> *(Ibid., p. 122)*

Mbiti notes that men over forty years of age participate in a third initiation that closely resembles joining a secret society. Initiates do not share any information about what happens during the initiation process and Mbiti says that even those men who become Christians are "unwilling to divulge what actually happens."

The Ndebele initiation rite of puberty for boys is mostly ceremonial. Boys undergo through a ritual washing off of the first emission of sperm, spend several days in the forests away from the community, and have dietary restrictions. "The idea of 'death and resurrection' is represented in the case of boys going to live for a few days in the forest."

The lives of African and enslaved African American boys and their descendants have evolved with the presence of the unconscious and archetypes. They have lived in circumstances of severe trauma through generations. They also have the potentiality of psychic energy and a spiritual dimension that exists for them through ancestral lineage.

As the idea of freedom from slavery took hold and became more infused with a collective archetypal energy this congealed into the Abolitionist movement. The black men and boys who joined this movement, and other ones like the maroon colonies, provided emotional sustenance to themselves as well as the enslaved Africanist communities of which they were members. How does the ancestral energy of African males who never left the continent of Africa and their captured descendants provide them with the energy to meet the challenges of today's contemporary life? We have learned a great deal more about not only the neuroscience of mirrored neurons but also the emotional connection that can exist between members of a family. Cultural groups have their own features and psychological markers that can now be accepted because it is obvious that environmental issues have also played a part in how we develop, not only as individuals, but also a group. The sons of enslaved women grew to be men leading Africanist people to sufficient consciousness to attain an identity that engaged the concept of freedom.

This engagement mirrored that of relationship within the self as exhibited by men such as Frederick Douglass and Nat Turner and also that which grew from a belief in the bonding with others that came from an African unconscious which held the kinship group as sacred and essential for survival.

10
THE FEMALE AFRICANIST BODY

A historical perspective

The history of the presence of Africanist women bodies in America began on a tragic note. It continued in this way for centuries. For example, in slavery, a way designed to protect African American unborn children who served as one main source of plantation profit, while punishing the pregnant mother, is described by Jacqueline Jones in *Labor of Love, Labor of Sorrow: Black Women, Work, and the Family, from Slavery to the Present*:

> One particular method of whipping pregnant slaves was used throughout the South: They were made to lie face down in a specially dug depression in the ground, a practice that provided simultaneously for the protection of the fetus and the abuse of its mother. Enslaved women's roles as workers and as childbearers came together in these trenches, these graves for the living, in southern plantation fields.
> *(2010, p. 19)*

When African women were first brought to America they entered the country as slaves to be used as labor for the economic success of the colonies. Early reports of the arrival of these women showed that they were usually treated no differently than the black men who came with them on slave ships, with the very important exception of sexual assault.

However, before the slave ships, what might have been the life experience, the bodily experience, of Africanist women? The history of African women indicates that prior to colonization, women had a distinctive and impressive role in the family and in the community, particularly as healers. The lineage of African women healers traveled to the New World and was a source of comfort and medical support for both slaves and their plantation owners.

Even before these times, in ancient time of queens, African women ruled kingdoms and were chiefs. Their bodies had been imaged and celebrated over centuries before reaching the American shores as chained slaves.

The African matriarchy appears to have ruled since before 15,000 BC in different countries throughout the continent. A major event that contributed to this change this was the continuing invasion of the southern part of the African continent by northern Muslim countries in the 12th and 13th centuries. Following these invasions, European colonization became the next major destabilizing traumatic event to take place in African countries. The historical existence of African matriarchal societies has been shown to appear in countries such as Egypt, Ghana, Angola and Nigeria. Both Egypt and Nigeria have rich histories that can be followed in terms of societal values and cultural mores. Egyptian society was ruled strictly by matrilineal family lines with all political power and wealth overseen by women.

In addition, both Egypt and Nigeria have recognizable archetypal histories that include goddesses, gods and mythologies that speak to their collective spiritual and religious practices. In the creation myth of Mawu (see below) one can see the goddess, the matriarchal line, the bringing of death by the masculine, and other features of the tradition of the African mother.

> Riding in the mouth of a great snake came Mawu to create the world, making mountains, rivers, and valleys along the snake's serpentine course. The better to view creation, she made a great fire in the sky, and added to the world elephants and lions, giraffes and wildebeests in great herds, bands of monkeys, as well as people. Her work accomplished, she sent the snake under the earth, where, coiled up, it would support the weight of the creation, and Mawu retired to the lofty jungle realm of heaven.
>
> Before long, the people began to fight among themselves, having forgotten that it was Mawu who had provided them not only with a world to live on, but, more important, with part of herself—the essence of life, their souls, a force called Sekpoli. To fight someone was thus to fight Mawu as well.
>
> Seeing all this turmoil, Mawu's daughters and granddaughters set out through the lands of Dahomey to remind people of the wisdom of Mawu and encountered an insolent braggart named Awe, who boasted that he was just as powerful as Mawu. Among his powers of music and magic, he, too, he blustered, could make life, and many people began to believe.
>
> To prove it, he threw three two balls of silk into the air and climbed up the threads through the clouds into the jungle of heaven, where he challenged Mawu, saying his powers were as great as hers. He chopped down a tree and carved on it all the features of a person. When he was finished, he stepped back and said, "I have created a person."
>
> Mawu observed the wooden figure lying on the ground. "How is it," she said, "that your person doesn't smile, doesn't walk, doesn't dance and chant in thanks to you? You should breathe Sekpoli into it, the essence of life." Awe

gulped an enormous breath of air and blew out so mightily that the jungle of heaven quivered as in a storm. But his person lay still and mute on the ground. Again, Awe gulped air and blew it out, so strongly that the person on the ground moved in the wind's path. But again it lay still and lifeless.

After two more attempts, Awe knew he was defeated and hung his head in shame. Only Mawu, he confessed, could make life. Only Mamu was wise. He was humbled and said he would return to the world below and explain this. But Mawu knew that Awe was at heart a charlatan and, once he returned to earth, would boast again. She made him a bowl of cereal to eat before his journey, into which she had put the seed of death.

Only when Awe had finished eating did he learn of the seed he had eaten and would carry back to earth. Mawu sent him off to explain that only Mawu could breathe the breath of life into people and, lest they value this gift lightly, could suck it out when she chose.

(Leeming, 1996, pp. 51–53)

African American women are descended not only from the strongest of those who could survive slavery but also from African women who owned, controlled and developed agricultural land on the African continent. The fact of the ownership of land in many African countries in pre-colonial times speaks to the overwhelming power of African American women to work under the conditions of slavery and produce economic success for white plantation owners in the days of slavery. The women who planted tobacco, rice and cotton had within their DNA and collective memory the remembrance of their female ancestors. It is no wonder that plantations thrived. It was of course not only the black bodies of women as we well know, but also those of men, children and even grandparents. But my focus here on the story of the wealthiest Africanist women who left Africa as the daughters of queens and arrived as captured slaves.

The plantation lands worked by these Africanist women would never belong to them, despite the promises made to them following the American Civil War— African Americans were promised forty acres and a mule to provide them with economic freedom. How bitter must have been the memory of those early women slaves who through stories had heard of the success of their African women ancestors. These ancestors, the ones who had not been brought into slavery but who had worked and owned their own fields and farms and supplied food to the people belonging to their towns and villages. There must have been stories because griots (storytellers) helped to transmit via stories the lives and experiences of the African people who came to America. The separation of the men and women who were to become slaves could not prevent the eventual integration of African practices based on regional and traditional rituals, healing and spiritual practices.

This is especially noticeable in the recorded linguistic history of the Gullah people off and on the coast of Georgia and South Carolina. This told of the lineage of Africanist women agriculturists who survived the Middle Passage and became realized in the slavery plantations throughout the South.

Bearing sorrow

One issue of the attempted invisibility of African Americans since American slavery has been the dual struggle contained within a racist structure of taking possession of the black body while making African Americans invisible. This has made for a very unique American bind. The purposeful intent of usage involving black bodies made it impossible to create African Americans as invisible. As a result, *African Americans had to take on the pretense of being invisible*. This showed itself in all the ways of racism affecting African Americans. No eye contact with whites, moving their bodies to the dirt or the street gutter, off the pavement when a white person approached. These were the "milder," intentionally shaming, social forms that racism took as regards the African American physical body.

The documented sexual fantasy, torture and rape of black women following their arrival in America made invisibility impossible, except as part of a racist imagination. There was an inherent problem in creating black women's bodies as unworthy of anything other thing than hard plantation labor while exploiting these same bodies for sexual pleasure.

This pleasure was in service of the plantation owner, overseer or any other white male who felt that he could claim power over African American women. These women could never fully claim their own bodies. In the most minimal manner, they could claim the suffering of carrying a child through pregnancy. But even here this was still not a complete claim since the child she was carrying could never fully belong to her, the mother. The visibility of a pregnant black mothering slave pointed to one essential possibility—that more children would be born into the plantation system.

The visibility of a pregnant black mothering slave pointed to the *denial* of invisibility of the black body, and its use as a mechanism for the increased frequency of black slavery, white racism, supremacy and economic power. The disempowerment of African American women as to the possession of their own bodies matched the historical empowerment of the black women in some African societies. These women were the descendants of queens and kings. When missionaries and European explorers came to the African continent they found African leaders—the descendants of these same kings and queens.

An African philosophical underpinning of the female body comes from traditional matriarchal narratives where women are the mothers who give and keep life. The proof of the truth of this statement is the contemporary challenge to Africans of how to allow women to claim true power through their lives as women. This would include even those women who do not bear children. Through centuries of belief it has been held within African societies that women are expected to procreate.

It is probably the reason for an underpinning within contemporary society that a woman does not merit respect in African society if she has not become a mother. This idea is dominant in the culture and has often found itself within the literature of different African societies. Literature is but one aspect of culture that shows the underpinning of this idea of the necessity of women to have children. The century-old rite of passage for entering adulthood through puberty rituals underscores the demand for women to produce children.

Imagine the disruption to the African female psyche as she saw her body and that of her female children without the sacred rites of passage that marked the entry into adulthood. Imagine the psychic and emotional suffering of the demand for the human body by those who had no understanding nor care to understand the feminine rituals of entering adulthood. Imagine the psychological trauma of losing touch with all that had belonged to you as an African woman anticipating marriage, bearing children with your husband, surrounded by his family and yours. Imagine this as you picked cotton from morning until night and then became the sexual object of any white man on the plantation who the slave owner designated. Imagine your pregnancy from rape. The eventual sale of the child. Imagine this.

The African American female body was lost to her upon embarking on the slave ship, even before she landed in America. The comparison of the physical life of African women as compared to their lives upon arriving in America bore no similarities with the exception of working on the land. This is the generalized version of the similarity.

The specific elements of what occurred were dramatically different. There was a very rare escape from having one's body used by men on the plantations. The powerlessness of women in these circumstances have been looked at historically with differing opinions. There are those who wrote about these early experiences of Africanist women slaves as being well cared for and brought to a soulful environment where they might have eventual heavenly salvation. I do believe that today we know this was a rationalization for the continuation of the sexual abuse of women and girls and the racist economic justification of slavery. The truth is more evidenced by the story of Sarah Baartman, a South African woman born circa 1789. Her more common name was Venus Hottentot, a name given to her after she arrived in England as a young adult. Baartman, it is believed, was intimidated against her will to come to England to be part of a circus. It is very likely that she had no idea of the purpose for which she had been specifically chosen. Once arriving Baartman was put on display for circus audience members to be seen as a show "freak." The reason for this was because of her body measurements—the size of her buttocks and breasts. The physical attributes of this African woman's body caused her to be virtually stolen from her homeland and shamelessly paraded in front of hundreds of spectators over the years.

Baartman was not the first Khoikhoi woman to be taken to Europe; many others were to follow. However, the plight of Baartman became symbolic because she was a symbol of the desecration of the Africanist female body. She was put on display in both England and Ireland after which time she traveled to Paris where she became ill and died. Following her time as a human circus "event," Baartman's remains—including her genitalia—were exhibited at the Museum of Man. This "exhibition" remained in place for over one hundred years. Though British Abolitionists protested against Baartman being displayed, they were unsuccessful in stopping the exhibition, even through a court trial. The failure to obtain her release reflected the enslavement of Africanist women bodies imprisoned on plantations. At the time of Baartman's death it would be another thirty-five years before the Emancipation Proclamation freed American slaves.

Body as narrative

In 1974, Donald Johanson and his team of paleontologists made the discovery of an early pre-homo sapiens skeleton fossil. These bones, found in Ethiopia, were said to have been the skeletal remains of a female more than three million years old. The scientists who made the discovery of this first ancestor named her Lucy. The eventual examinations and tests carried out on Lucy showed that she was indeed the oldest representation of early human existence. She was found in Africa.

The respect given to ancestors by Africanist people lives deep within the Africanist psyche and the body. Africans saw no separation between the mind and the body. When Jung references participation mystique in his discussion of the consciousness of Africans he is not mistaken in his recognition of such a possible state of consciousness. His error is in applying only a negative theory related to a lack of potential intellectual growth and individuation for Africanist individuals at the conclusion of his study.

He does not see them as capable of being individuals—only joined in a lower level of consciousness noted as *participation mystique*. Jung both accepted this state of consciousness as something Europeans had lost and which had value while at the same time criticizing Africans for having a lower level of consciousness due to it. There can be no mistake. This was a racial commentary made in a sociological frame useful to building a theory of consciousness.

The philosophical belief of Africanist people is that there is no separation of mind and body. The body remembers long after the mind has forgotten what it has seen or heard. The body tells a story. This is actually a position that has become more in evidence in recent times as we see the development of somatic psychology as an area of professional interest and study among psychologists.

The African diaspora female body tells her own story. It is one characterized by centuries-long trauma. As Lucy appeared into our 20th-century life, as we considered the existence of the *first* female humanoid, the undercurrent of that time had existed for centuries. An almost parallel circumstance that continued as a part of the racial undercurrent was the persecution of African diaspora women in many forms. One of these forms included the prosecution of these women. Dorothy Roberts states the following in her preface to *Killing the Black Body: Race, Reproduction and the Meaning of Liberty*:

> In the late 1980s, I began to notice news stories about prosecutions of women for using drugs while pregnant. District attorneys across the country concocted an assortment of charges to punish them for fetal crimes—child neglect, distribution of drugs to a minor, assault with a deadly weapon, and attempted

murder. How did a public health problem become a criminal justice matter to be solved by locking up women instead of providing them with better health care? I was sure of three things about the prosecutions: they primarily targeted Black women, they punished these women for having babies, and they were a form of both race and gender oppression.

(2017, p. vi)

As we consider the history of Africanist women bodies, there is a tension—an anxious gaze that anticipates that a negative life-threatening social event that will occur. We might say that this is the post-traumatic effect of slavery. It could be the constellation of a racial complex or it might just be living in a daily conscious state of anticipatory fear in service to human survival or perhaps all of these things. By whatever name or description, we know that they survive in our racialized American psyche. Since leaving the African continent enslaved, the status of African diaspora women has been marked with horror, a profound lack of compassion and a racist orientation that has continued into the 21st century. In *Sister Citizen: Shame, Stereotypes, and Black Women in America*, Melissa V. Harris Perry states:

> Welfare policy is intimately linked in the American imagination with black women's sexuality. Political scientist Martin Gilens shows that white American opposition to welfare results from whites' fixed beliefs that the system supports unworthy black people who lack a suitable work ethic. Central to this opposition is a belief that black women do no appropriately control their fertility, that they have sex with multiple partners, producing children who must be cared or through tax-supported social welfare programs …. The depiction of black women as sexually insatiable breeders suits a slaveholding society that profits from black women's fertility. *But for a shrinking postmodern state, black women's assumed lasciviousness and rampant reproduction are threatening.* Therefore throughout the twentieth century the state employed involuntary sterilization, pressure to submit to long-term birth control, and restriction of state benefits for large families as a way to control black women's reproduction. The myth of a plantation Jezebel can be deployed to limit today's welfare-dependent mother.
>
> It is not just a matter of distorted perceptions; this misrecognition can be used to punish African American women through policy.
>
> *(2011, pp. 67–68; emphasis added)*

The black racial complex and the resulting anxieties of white Americans can create any variation of imaginative roles for African American women. We have witnessed the development of these stereotypes over the years. Some have changed form—like the mammy who was an always available nurse maid and housekeeper—while in the post-slavery era of the 21st century the stereotype of the angry, aggressive, over-sexed welfare mother has been created. However, we may look at these fantasized images of African diaspora women and realize that those of this lineage carry not only the slavery-era DNA of survival but also the pre-colonial energy and empowerment of Africanist women. In the oppositional effort to make us forget ourselves and add to our own invisibility, we must always engage in the affirmative effort to remember and bring into consciousness the nature of survival—the necessity of remembering what our bodies tell us; to harness the survivalist energy of our ancestors who lived through slavery and beyond. For African diaspora women the true work is recalling the Africanist's body story that developed from African queens and stories of beauty from the goddess Oshun. This story is not the racially inspired false one which makes the black body over-sexed and in need of sterilization, over-productive, and in need of oppression, or over-exotic and in need of white sanitization. Memory recall can be engaged to help the body to heal through a recollection of what the body already knows. If archetypally we are able to bring forth the grief of slavery's intergenerational trauma, our work is to bring forth the storied memory of who we were prior to colonization.

Today there is no economic use for African American women's bodies in the reproduction system of slave-breeding. Within the American racial psyche is the changed story of how Africanist women use their bodies to steal from the welfare system. There is a gross irony in this turn of events, in this thinking that *blames* the female victim. There is no forgetting because the body does not forget. The archetypal energy of the ancestors and the archetypes themselves all join in pushing recollection when the ego desires only restful peace. But for those who made the passage across the waters and their descendants who survived centuries of slavery, the spirit of recall does not disappear. There can only be a profound archetypal recollection and prayers that turns the egregious into true grief that permits healing of mind and body.

The first freedom

Once the American Civil War ended, all Americans, both white and black, were forced to face their differences but this time African Americans wore the face of freedom. Many in the tradition of Quakers, Abolitionists and others open to racial equality were still fearful of black revenge and retaliation for all the years of slavery. Following the Civil War anxieties and tensions were high due to white Southern rage at having lost the war. Vigilante groups emerged from the darkness carrying fire and burning crosses. Jim Crow laws began to surface in all parts of the South. Segregation became the eventual Southern response to the North having won the war and freed men, women and children out of bondage.

This first freedom for African Americans coming out of slavery was that of the body. I can barely imagine the release, the ecstasy of claiming the body after decades, centuries of having it belong to others. The mental preparation for those born into slavery had already begun within the last fifty years before the Emancipation Proclamation. In my fantasy, I can picture the jubilation of some of my own ancestors knowing that they could have possession of their bodies—no more overseers, no near starvation, no more forced labor from morning until night.

The experience of freeing the body for African American women had its own signifier that meant freedom from a guarantee of rape and all forms of sexual assault without consequence. This freedom of the body meant escape from serving as a mothering slave for countless children that could all be taken, leaving you always a breeder of children—never a mother. It must be noted, Emancipation did not put an end to sexual assault on black women and lynching replaced legal plantation torture.

This first freedom of the body followed years of slavery with all of its torture as was described in oral slave narratives following emancipation. Here is one account by a former slave:

> My marster had a barrel, with nails drove in it, that he would put you in when he couldn't think of nothin' else mean enough to do. He would put you in this barrel and roll it down a hill. When you got out you would be in a bad fix, but he didn't care. Sometimes he rolled the barrel in the river and drowned his slaves.
>
> *(Mellon, 1988, p. 247)*

Here is another brief account by a former young African American soldier:

> When I went to the War, I was turning seventeen. I was in the Battle of Nashville, when we whipped old (General) Hood. I went to see my mistress on my furlough, and she was glad to see me. She said, "You remember when you were sick and I had to bring you to the house and nurse you?" And I told her, "Yes'm, I remember". And she said, "And now, you are fighting me!" I said, No'm, I aint't fighting you. I'm fighting to get free."
>
> *(Ibid., p. 339)*

Following the first freedom of the body came the freedom of the mind. I imagine that this was just as much a relief as finally having the body freed from slavery. During all the years immediately following the passage of the 13th Amendment abolishing slavery in America, the African American collective mind was not only traumatized from all the decades and centuries of slavery but also the event of freedom itself which saw the rise of white nationalism. A former slave, Hester Norton, remembers: "I was pow'ful glad when I wuz freed. One thing they did wuz to whitewash de bullwhip and hang it on de side of de house" (Mellon, 1988, p. 354). I believe that a third freedom for African Americans following emancipation was freedom of the spirit, but it took almost another fifty years for it to be realized through the work of Dr. Martin Luther King.

The spiritual songs that had been sung throughout all the years of plantation life had provided an emotional salve and a salvation to millions. These same spiritual songs helped African Americans to move into post-war Reconstruction and the beginning of the 20th century. However, the freedom that had been hoped for in the previous forty years did not come to fruition. Segregation only grew stronger as the forces of the Abolitionist movement, the Freedman's Bureau and the number of African Americans in Congress became almost non-existent.

The first half of the 20th century saw two world wars. African Americans served in both of these wars in segregated units. In the same way that spirituals had carried African Americans through the slavery era, so did the blues and later gospel carry us through the years of lynching, Jim Crow and the Ku Klux Klan. I think it took and continues to take a significant level of strength and determination to survive and for the spirit to remain alive and not to be completely broken following centuries of cruel and inhumane torture such as that experienced by African Americans. Women who had been active in a movement to *steal away* and end slavery were in the forefront of the push to gain rights for protecting their bodies and their children following the Emancipation Proclamation.

When Dr. Martin Luther King began protesting for African American civil liberties in 1956, he was to become the first hero emerging since the Civil War with the exception of Marcus Garvey who embodied the spirit of freedom that had been promised and fought for but never realized. His oratory was inspiring and rose to the heights of evangelical uplifting for African Americans. Dr. King's appearance at the end of the 1950s ushered in a new spirit that would lift and carry African Americans until the voice of Malcolm X and the Black Power movement took possession of body, mind and spirit. The coming together of these three aspects of the African American psyche infused members of this community and furthered an empowerment of a positive black consciousness that had not been fully realized since the end of slavery. This allowed for the emergence of not only the history of black Americans told from their point of view, but also for the initiation of a dialogue in which African Americans could speak for themselves and define their own psychological selves without interpretation of a white Other.

11

MIRROR AS SYMBOL

> The glory of the day was in her face,
> The beauty of the night was in her eyes.
> And over all her loveliness, the grace
> Of Morning blushing in the early skies.
> *James Weldon Johnson (1871–1938)*

Mami Wata is a Nigerian goddess whose influence has spread as far as South America, brought by the African diaspora. Her name means Mother Water with an etymology of truth, wisdom and water. Her attributes are snake, water and objects of the rivers and the seas. The development of the goddess Mami from ancient Babylonian times has reached through the centuries into Ethiopian and Egyptian mythology. In her essence as Mother Water she is the mother of healing, and the protector of mothers and children.

In Western mythology, Mami, or the mermaid Siren, is often portrayed as a seductress who lured men to their deaths or inflicted some other form of punishment. In African mythology, this goddess has evolved into one who provides a lineage of seers, prophetesses, orators and healers. Mami evolved in African mythology to join a group of water deities who included Isis. As a water goddess Mami is represented with a mirror which she holds to her face giving her own reflection. This is an African tradition whereby as the protector of children and mothers, she holds a mirror to her face to reflect all that she is and can give to her followers—women, men and children.

According to Ami Ronnberg in *The Book of Symbols: Reflections on Archetypal Images*:

> The use of the mirror as an attribute of beauty, knowledge, wisdom and a giving return reflection has been present in most societies from the beginning of time. Mirrors have always existed. Before the use of metal, they were the

reflections on the waters collected in the earth's indentations. Early peoples believed that in such reflections the soul element could be perceived and even today the fantasy persists that the mirror can steal one's soul. The association of the mirror with the essential nature of a thing is carried in the ancient Egyptian hieroglyph for life, the ankh, which was also one of the words for mirror. The mirror represented the solar disk as the source of light that contained life's essence. Mirrors were placed in burial chambers and were also cult objects in the worship of Hathor, goddess of abundance, joy, music, dance, cosmetics and self-beautification, which brought one into harmony with the divine.

(2010, p. 590)

The mirror of Mami Wata can itself act as a divine object reflecting the potential healing energy for mothers and their children. The creation myth of Mami contained in Tablet 1 (a Sumerian 18th century BC writing tablet) of the epic king Atrahasis shows that at the gods' request the goddess created man so that he could shoulder the gods' burdens and problems. Man was to become the scapegoat of the gods. In turn, man, in his own way, has shifted the weight of life's burdens onto others.

The involvement of Mami in the original myth before its evolution to Mami Wata points to a shift from divine to human. It also shows the flow of archetypal energy that shifts the balance of psychic power. This power coming through the Mami archetypal lineage as reflected in the mirror of the divine transfers power to womankind. What is possible for women in the goddess/archetypal lineage from one who holds the mirror? How can we use such a question to redirect consciousness towards influencing the archetypes? I will use a narrative from Japanese culture to illustrate a connection between spirituality, the mirror and the unconscious.

The following narrative is a reflection of an aspect of my own thoughts and engagement regarding intertwining sections of human consciousness of Buddhism, Jungian psychology and mythological amplification of the mirror.

Kensho: The Mirror of Self-Reflection

Thus have I heard. On one occasion the Blessed One was living at Rajagaha in the Bamboo Grove, the Squirrels's Sanctuary. Now on that occasion the venerable Rahula was living at Ambalatthika. Then when it was evening, the Blessed one rose from meditation and went to the venerable Rahula at Ambalatthika. The venerable Rahula saw the Blessed One coming in the distance and made a seat ready and set out water for washing the feet. The Blessed One sat down on the seat made ready and washed his feet. The venerable Rahula paid homage to him and sat down at one side.

The above words describe the opening passage of the *Ambalatthikarahulovada Sutta* 61, more commonly known as "Advice to Rahula at Ambalatthika" from *The Middle Length Discourses of the Buddha*. Rahula was the Buddha's son whom he left soon after birth. When Rahula was nine years old, some texts say seven, he went in search of his father who had by then become an enlightened teacher traveling to different parts of India.

> What do you think, Rahula? What is the purpose of a mirror?
> For the purpose of reflection, venerable sir.
> So too, Rahula, an action with the body should be done after repeated reflection: an action by speech should be done after repeated reflection; an action by mind should be done after repeated reflection.
> (Nanamoli, B. and Bodhi, B. (trans.) 2005, p. 523, (p. 414), paras 1, 2)

Each day most of us look in a mirror, seeing ourselves reflected. Usually it is upon rising—the best time to see ourselves before we put on the mask of persona and the colors which separate us from those we meet in the world. It is fitting that the first face we meet should be our own. This is the training of becoming a Jungian analyst. We must first meet ourselves in personal analysis which prepares us to meet an Other—the patient. However, in writing this, I am reminded that in Buddhism, there is no Other, only the Self meeting the Self in what looks like otherness.

> Ruhula, when you wish to do an action with the body, you should reflect upon that same bodily action thus: 'Would this action that I wish to do with the body lead to my own affliction, or to the affliction of others, or to the affliction of both?'
> Also, Rahula while you are doing an action with the body, you should reflect upon that same bodily action thus: 'Does this action that I am doing with the body lead to my own affliction, or to the affliction of others, or to the affliction of both?'
> Also, Rahula, after you have done an action with the body, you should reflect upon that same bodily action thus: 'Did this action that I did with the body lead to my own affliction, or to the affliction of others, or to the affliction of both?'
> (2005, pp. 524–525, (415–416), paras 9, 10, 11)

In this teaching to his son, the Buddha touches not just on reflection of the body but also on speech and the mind. He tells his son that like the mirror he must reflect on action of the body, speech and the mind, before, during and after such actions are taken. It is important to note that Rahula is told to *first* reflect upon himself and then others. He must first see if he has caused himself pain or affliction then look to others. This Buddhist teaching reminds us that we are the first to look at ourselves. Our responsibility is first to gaze at our own reflection before we begin the mirroring work with others. The Buddha concludes his teaching to Rahula with the following:

> Therefore, Rahula, you should train thus: "We will purify our bodily action, our verbal action, and our mental action by repeatedly reflecting upon them."
> (2005, p. 526, (420), para. 18)

The Buddha's word 'train' provides us with the direction in which to focus the mind, preparing ourselves to reflect on all that we do before, during and after our actions. It is insufficient to focus on our actions just during one phase; we are required to consider ourselves and our actions before, during and after they have taken place. This bringing into consciousness of our body, speech and mind is another way of viewing the moment to moment observation of Self as in observing the breath during zazen sitting practice.

How can we mirror ourselves in ways that do not merely gratify the ego? In Jungian work, we presuppose the necessary strengthening of the ego in preparation for a journey to the unconscious. However, too much egoic fortitude in service only to the ego makes for a very difficult or an incomplete journey. In achieving a balance between ego strength and a willingness to see into our shadow material, we must develop a bridging vision which can consistently hold dismantling and repair. The personal work of both Buddhism and analytical psychology requires such a vision. In the mirrored effect of continuous viewing, one can see the blemishes of ego and hopefully through practice, clean and polish the mirror. This is the work of a lifetime.

In *Projection and Re-Collection of the Soul in Jungian Psychology*, Marie-Louise von Franz, discusses the beginning of reflection in human consciousness. She agrees with Jung's belief that before humans developed myths, they were capable of what she terms "momentary flashes of consciousness." The latter were performed in rituals as impulsive acts. Over time, these impulses became organized within the ego as personal experiences. Von Franz says further of these "flashes":

> They, too, were originally represented in symbolic form and given a ritual application in the shape of glittering small stones, or other shiny mirror-like objects to which were subscribed the power to drive away spirits .... Even when we attempt, through indirect conclusions, to know not the external world but the nature of the objective psyche, that is of the unconscious, we mirror it in our ego-consciousness.
>
> *(1980, p. 179)*

In the section entitled "Fourfold Mirroring," von Franz discusses four ways in which psychic mirroring occurs in human beings. These intersections occur between ego and Self mirroring each other along with the mirroring exchange between matter and the collective unconscious. Von Franz states:

> Therefore when the ego follows the signals given in dreams, it is helping the Self attain realization in time and space. It is then "mirroring" the Self by lifting it out of its unconscious, merely potential existence, into the clarity of ego consciousness.
>
> *(1980, pp. 187–188)*

Von Franz notes two of Jung's own dreams from his autobiography. Each one of these dreams shows the mirror-image relations between ego and Self. In one dream, Jung sees a flying saucer overhead in the sky. In the second dream, discussed in *Memories, Dreams, Reflections*, Jung believes that he is being "imagined" by a yogi:

> I had dreamed once before of the problem of the Self and the ego. In that earlier dream I was on a hiking trip. I was walking along a little road through a hilly landscape; the sun was shining and I had a wide view in all directions. Then I came to a small wayside chapel. The door was ajar, and I went in. To my surprise there was no image of the Virgin on the altar, and no crucifix either, but only a wonderful flower arrangement. But then I saw that on the floor in front of the altar, facing me, sat a yogi—in lotus posture, in deep meditation. When I looked at him more closely, I realized that he had my face. I started in profound fright, and awoke with the thought: "Aha, so he is the one who is meditating me. He has a dream, and I am it." I knew that when he awakened, I would no longer be.
>
> *(1973, p. 323)*

In both dreams, Jung finds that the Self has created him (ego) and placed him in a reality which is in alignment with the Self's stance. Von Franz alleges that the Self is the "Other" within each individual's existence. However, it is also the ego, since it is from the Self projecting/mirroring that we can assume identity.

If we believe that inside each of us exists our own "Other," then we are more likely to initiate and engage in doing the inner work that is necessary for deepening our lives. We would assume the exchange between ego and Self to be a necessity, as much as taking each next breath. We can see from von Franz's illustration that both ego and Self are required. Each one serves our development in a different way and yet gives us a sense of psychic wholeness. When this is unavailable, we experience psychic breaks—mental, or spiritual—which leave us without connectedness to ourselves, others or our material world. A major avenue of connection to our cultural collective has evolved through the stories we hear and tell by way of our mythology, legends and fairy tales.

Myths and legends

In Japanese culture, many of the myths and legends originated in the Shinto religion which preceded the introduction of Buddhism into Japan. The original mythology is recorded in the Kojiki and the Nihongi Texts. The writing thereof was commanded by Emperor Temmi (673–686 CE in order to create a permanent historical record of Japan's mythology and the development of its' monarchy.

Jung, in one of his many discussions concerning mythology, states, "Myths and fairy tales give expression to unconscious processes, and their retelling causes these processes to come alive again and be recollected, thereby re-establishing the connection between conscious and unconscious" (CW9ii, para. 280). We can see from Jung's statement that mythology was considered by him to be an important avenue of communication for relationship between ego and self as experienced by each new generation.

The history of the mirror as symbol in Japan is given below:

> Japanese mythology suggests that the original "spirit-body" was that of Amaterasu, the Sun Goddess, who gave a circular mirror to her grandson, Ninigi, when he descended to earth. It had been used previously in an elaborate ruse to lure her out of a cave in which she was hiding. Her absence had plunged the world into darkness, and to tempt her out she was told that there was another goddess as beautiful as herself. The mirror was held up so that when she peeked out she was greeted by her own radiance, and the momentary hesitation allowed a rope to be tied across the cave entrance so as to prevent her from re-entering. Sunlight was restored to the world.
>
> *(www.greenshinto.com)*

Antique Japanese mirrors were made so that the glass that reflects the face also allows for the images painted on the back of the glass to show through in the reflection. In viewing oneself individuals were allowed to see a deeper image. The purpose of the mirror is to show us as we are without falsehoods or deceits. A Japanese proverb attributed to the mirror is "When the mirror is dim, the soul is unclean." The god Izangi, in giving his children the mirrors and admonishing them to use these reflective tools, sets the example for humans as to how we are to see and reflect upon ourselves—with a pure spirit. There are times however, when this may seem impossible.

> There is a story of a wrestler who was accustomed to wear as an ornament on his forehead a precious stone. One time when he was wrestling the stone was crushed into the flesh of his forehead. He thought he had lost the gem and went to a surgeon to have the wound dressed. When the surgeon came to dress the wound he found the gem embedded in the flesh and covered over with blood and dirt. He held up a mirror and showed the stone to the wrestler.
>
> *(American Buddhist Academy, 1966, pp. 73–74)*

In this story, the wrestler believes that he has lost the stone, something of immense value to him. However, the stone has only been covered by blood and dirt. This story is about retaining belief in what we think that we have lost, that which is sacred to us—the precious jewel of the Self. When the wrestler is face to face with himself again, he is able to see the stone. Only when he faces himself in the mirror, and receives a cleansing, is he then able to see the stone. Through the mirror we are able to see that which is precious to us—our own nature, including the psychological dirt which covers us. The truth of the reflected image is that it cannot lie. A mirror forces the viewer to see for himself/herself all that is visible and, in the case of antique Japanese mirrors, also what lies behind the glass. Persona is seen as well as what lies behind it.

> The importance of the mirror is its symbol as soul. In Japanese culture, it is believed that what appears in the glass is a direct reflection of the individual's soul. Over time, the mirror begins to take on the traits and attributes of its owner as a result of the archetypal energy at rests behind the glass surface as the unconscious encompasses the ego.
>
> (Brewster, 2012, pp. 51–57)

The mother is the first human mirror that reflects who we are and is a major influence on who we are to become as adults. In the sacred and spiritual space that exists between mother and child grows a bond that is reflective of the care, emotions and physical attunement resonating with both of them. Once this connection is made it is unlikely that any separation will cause it to break even in the absence of the mother. The presence of the mother is mythological because, as Jung says, the biological mother represents all the mothers who have ever come before, going all the way back to the goddess-archetype mother.

Mothering slaves embodied the potentiality of this goddess-mother and gave it as an inheritance to their daughters. This is the potential that became a realized force of energy as the culture of African diaspora required this energy in response to slavery and then freedom. The aunts and grandmothers who for centuries had taken care of the children of mothering slaves, in the absence of biological mothers, inherited positive attributes as women who survived slavery and achieved success, power and influence—for themselves and their communities by assuring the continued survival of their cultural collective.

12

INFLUENCING THE ARCHETYPE

In his discussion of the archetype Jung describes Hitler's racial attacks on Jewish people prior to the Second World War. I find it a unique experience to read Jung's words in light of our American political collective events that have taken place since the presidential election of 2016. Jung states:

> Since neuroses are in most cases not just private concerns, but *social* phenomena, we must assume that archetypes are constellated in these cases too. The archetype corresponding to the situation is activated and as a result those explosive and dangerous forces hidden in the archetype come into action, frequently with unpredictable consequences. There is no lunacy people under the domination of an archetype will not fall a prey to. If thirty years ago anyone had dared to predict that our psychological development was tending towards a revival of the medieval persecutions of the Jews, that Europe would again tremble before the Roman fasces and the tramp of legions, that people would once more give the Roman salute, as two thousand years ago and that instead of the Christian Cross an archaic swastika would lure on millions of warriors ready for death— why, that man would have been hooted at as a mystical fool. And today?
>
> *(CW9i, para. 98; emphasis in the original)*

Jung's words would appear to confirm the existence of the archetypes and their influence on the individual as well as the collective. Presently, we do not have "millions of warriors ready for death" among our American white nationalist population, but there are many thousands who are. They have their swastika symbols and they still harbor a negative bias against Jews and African Americans. Jung presented his lecture containing the above reference in 1936.

Some eight decades later we are facing a constitutional and democratic crisis as American citizens of color come under attack through the political sway of the current government Administration. We have had our Charlottesville. We have had the violent protests to keep Confederate statues standing which symbolize the racism of Jim Crow in post-Civil War America. With all of this we have witnessed the flying of the swastika and heard the chants of men and women marching against Jews. This is not Jung's 1936, this is our 21st century—our today.

I have used Jung's descriptive words in connection with the archetypes and social phenomena, because *Archetypal Grief: Slavery's Legacy of Intergenerational Child Loss* speaks directly to the event of African American persecution under slavery—a social phenomenon. Jung spoke many times about the German Holocaust that killed millions of Jewish people. It has been necessary for those of the generations following him remember and address the African Holocaust and cultural trauma of the African diaspora. In using Jungian psychology to address this intergeneration trauma I believe that I can borrow with reliability Jung's concept of the archetypes. It would be unlikely and impossible to express support of some of Jung's ideas regarding his interpretation of the collective unconscious. This is particularly true when he discusses certain racial factors specific to Africanist people. In his attempt to confirm his theory of the collective unconscious, racial ideas aligned themselves with racism. (Brewster, 2017) However, when Jung speaks of the nature of human consciousness and the existence of archetypal patterns and energy of psyche, I can accept his conceptualization.

Jean Knox, George Hogenson and others interested in Jung's archetypes and the collective unconscious have begun to explore the possibility of a non-classical Jungian nature of the archetypes. This difference relates more to the archetypes as action patterns that do not necessarily originate from an unconscious place but rather are a result of neurobiological factors such as mirror neurons, the social environment and species typical behaviors. In his paper entitled "Archetypes as Action Patterns", George Hogenson states the following in his discussion of analytical psychology and mirror neurons:

> What we have in the theory of archetypes, therefore, is a combination of features that include ways of knowing the world (patterns of apprehension and intuition—a specific subset, it seems, of ways of acting in the world), patterns of behavior, and affective states that accompany these intuitions and patterns of behavior, and finally, a notion of the image that appears to go beyond our common sense notion of the image as imply a picture or representation of some other state of affairs. The question that arises in the context of this meeting is what relationship these aspects of Jung's theory have to the discovery of mirror neurons.
>
> *(2009, p. 327)*

As we extend our knowledge regarding our cognitive, spiritual and conscious selves, we have the possibility for deepening ourselves in relationship. The most recent conversations regarding the epigenetics and mirror neurons and even attachment theory give Jungian psychology further avenues of exploration for understanding our nature in a picture of wholeness rather than divided into mind and body. In their discussion of human development in terms of cognition and behavior, Esther Thelen and Linda B. Smith, authors of *A Dynamic Systems Approach to the Development of Cognition and Action*, discern through their own studies that we as humans are actually developing even as they as researchers study human development.

Observer and participant are not separate. Each is affected by the presence of the other. I find this to be very similar to the nature of being with another in depth psychological work. We must be in touch or nothing happens in the development of relationship. Human knowledge and growth does not stop at any point. We continue to develop because we are alive. We are in an evolutionary process. Thelen and Smith say that their deepened understanding of human development has been acquired through their studies and it has become known to them as *process and change* (1996, p. 341) Our increased knowledge is based on involvement and relationship to the immediacy of living—we learn as we live and adapt accordingly. Jung has spoken about adaption as necessary throughout the course of a life. When we do not adapt we find ourselves misaligned with our core Self. This misalignment between ego and archetype shows itself in greater neurotic emotional suffering. I believe that this is one way to look at our human consciousness in relationship with that which is divine.

Due to acquired scientific studies over the past twenty years regarding how we as humans respond to one another based on mirror neurons, specified typical behaviors and epigenetics, it becomes easier to say that we imitate, learn and develop from one another in a variety of ways that include emotional learning. My interest is focused on emotional states, especially grief. In his reference to mirror neurons Hogensen, a Jungian analyst, brings to our attention the relationship between the archetypal and neurology. It really does open up our interests in questions regarding how we have come to accept and view the archetypes. Jean Knox has shown through her own writing the differing models she says Jung formulated for defining the archetypes. She lists these models as:

(1) Biological entities in the form of information which is hardwired in the genes, providing a set of instructions to the mind as well as to the body;
(2) Organizing mental frameworks of an abstract nature, a set of rules or instruction but with no symbolic or representational content, so they are never directly experienced;
(3) Core meanings which do contain representational content and which therefore provide a central symbolic significance to our experience;
(4) Metaphysical entities which are eternal and are therefore independent of the body.

(2012, p. 24)

As Knox continues her discussion of Jung and his models for the archetypes she argues that Jung did not realize that his models were "incompatible." Knox says,

"The evidence now available to us from contemporary cognitive science research would suggest that Jung was trying to reconcile models which are incompatible with each other in relation to the structures of the human psyche" (2012, p. 24). If we accept Jung's idea of "biological entities .... hardwired in the genes" containing information, we see more contemporary studies which connect this through studies of the brain in laboratory animal and human studies (ibid.). The work initiated by John Bowlby on attachment and mother-child relationships has been revisited by way of neuroscience studies. Jaak Panksepp and Lucy Biven in *The Archeology of Mind: Neuroevolutionary Origins of Human Emotions*, remind us:

> Only in recent years have neuroscientists been able to translate attachment theory into concrete changes that happen in the brain. Neuroscientists understand these brain changes in terms of epigenesist-gene expression that takes place as the result of experience .... Epigenesis involves experience-dependent gene expression; it is the gene expression that happens after birth as a result of the child's experiences in the world .... so when a previously dormant gene is expressed in particular brain circuits, it can produce proteins and neuropeptide that the brain cells have not previously produced. Many of these aroused neurochemical pathways surely modify affect BrainMind functions. Thus, we see how epigenetic processes can influence emotional behaviors and feelings.
>
> *(2012, p. 342)*

My own interest in understanding what I have labeled archetypal grief comes from the development of the transference of the quality and essence of emotion—grief with an underpinning of trauma from mother to child. Research suggests that if a mother is depressed and consequently unresponsive to her infant, one sees abnormalities in the child's behavior as well as its brain organization (Meaney, 2002; Tronick, 1986).

I believe that the intergenerational trauma of slavery and post-slavery events heavily influenced the psychological, physical and emotional lives of enslaved mothers and their children. I would suggest that current research studies point to genetic factors as well as the environment in understanding how we are to view trauma and parent-child relations. One of my questions concerns the intergeneration passing-on of grief and though apparently biological in one way, what of the other aspect of the archetypal? In looking at the physiological results to brain function of trauma—whether that of the absence of continuous good mothering or the visual imagery of frequent violence, it is more apparent that there is a relationship of the transference of genetic material which can actually become stronger over time *and* generations affecting the mental status of individuals. There are a set of instructions which would seem to inform us how we learn and how we live within a given environment. Can we call this archetypal? Perhaps we can. Can we relate this to the metaphysical of which Jung so often spoke? Perhaps we can. The acceptance or rejection of the idea of what is archetypal and what is not can be objective as well as subjective.

Why is it not possible to do away with divisions of the archetype and have a consolidation viewpoint? This follows Jung's way of studying the collective unconscious and his manner of bringing into a form—though at times not cleanly linear—the richness of varying ideas of being. His studies of Gnosticism, alchemy, Christianity, dreams and other ways in which he explored human consciousness provides an example of how we might view and define the archetypes. In their Epilogue Thelen and Smith state the following:

> In this book, we have argued that progress in understanding is not well served by the old dualistic thinking: structure vs. function, nature vs. nurture, brain vs. behavior, perception vs. cognition, mind vs. body, competence vs. performance, learning vs. development. What we have substituted instead is an approach that considers dynamics at all levels, where continuity and change can be accommodated under a single theoretical umbrella and where the dualistic boundaries are erased.
>
> *(1996, p. 341)*

How might it look to have an understanding of archetypes as part of the mystery of our human consciousness touched by something which is divine? Mystics have proven that we do not need a system to enter into a relationship with the divine. The power of Jung's various avenues that he traveled to come to his theory of the archetypes supports all of the ways in which we can have an experience of something outside of the range of daily personal unconscious activities. Our ability to add epigenetics to consideration of the archetypes adds and confirms Jung's own idea of genetics and culture (environment), the influence of the "dress" of culture to what can emerge as archetypal. It is important, I believe, as we gain more information to what we know of human development to strive for a gathering of knowledge. Metaphysics and biology do not have to be opposites in our growing understanding of ourselves as both human and spiritual beings.

When thinking of the metaphysical and transcendent nature of an archetype there is an experiential basis for a belief in archetypes as representing the divine. In religions and spiritual practices all over the world, humans believe in something greater than themselves which transcends the ego and gives numinous experiences. It could be said that one must take this on faith.

The discussion of mirror neurons is the primary topic in *Mirror in the Brain: How our minds share actions and emotions* by Giacomo Rizzolatti and Corrado Sinigaglia. The authors provide detailed evidence of their studies of how due to the mirroring quality of brain neurons we are able to interact with other human beings in a way of imitation that can be physical as well as emotional. This theory of mirror neurons and their functioning confirmed how within the clinical setting, the transference, therapeutic alliance and the quality of the work is influenced by the mutuality of relating between therapist and patient.

We have known about the transference, Jung's words about the need for the chemical reaction between patient and analyst and with the introduction of mirror neurons we could understand even more from a broader perspective. We could ask ourselves about the possible relationship between organic imaging of the brain and what might be possible from the unconscious. This would not be where all we see is produced by what we think we know, but rather from what we do not know—that place of discovery in which we live, and which creates that which we cannot know only through ego. How do we come to know what we do know from an unconscious place/space?

For many of African descent this unknowing returns to a place of the spiritual.

> According to African peoples, man lives in a religious universe, so that natural phenomena and objects are intimately associated with God. They not only originate from Him but also bear witness to Him. Man's understanding of God is strongly coloured by the universe of which man is himself a part. Man sees in the universe not only the imprint but the reflection of God; and whether that image is marred or clearly focused and defined, it is nevertheless an image of God, the only image known in traditional African societies .... Some of the matriarchal societies, like the Ovambo and southern Nuba, conceive or speak of God as "Mother," which conveys the same attributes as those who consider Him as "Father." The image of Mother also carries with it the idea of cherishing and nursing, and it is used even in patriarchal societies.
>
> *(Mbiti, 1989, pp. 48–49)*

All societies have religion that has grown from the earliest spiritual practices known to humankind. The matriarchal societies of the Mother, Buddhism, Taoism, Christianity—all arose because of a need in the human being for a connection with something beyond the ego. The need for a connection with the divine has been evidenced for thousands of years through rituals that recognize rites of passage. These rituals acknowledge the "passage" of a human experience that engages the divine—and vice versa. The exchange of energy, sometimes named the numinous when received by human beings, is life-altering. In this book, *Archetypal Grief*, I have sought to find a deeper understanding of the emotional impact of grief on intertwining generations of mothering slaves and their descendants. In seeking to find a more depthful location, I have remembered and thought about myself as a descendant of a mothering slave. I am not separate from the spiritual and biological ties that bind my ancestors. I know from historical factors about their spiritual beliefs and practices. I accept that there are limitations on how much I can conceive based only on the biological conditions of my brain. I would not assume that I am only a thinking mind without connection to every other living thing visible and invisible.

In this type of relationship, I also accept that archetypes can exist as patterns that are influential in my life, my cultural collective and the broader collective at large. In this acceptance I acknowledge that societal change, madness and "lunancy" do occur. The quotation from Jung at the beginning of this chapter addresses the influence that archetypes can have over us on an individual as well as a collective level. The racial complex, which I believe has as a center the shadow archetype of racism, without conscious effort to interact with it, forces us to act out aggression and violence against one another based on *othering*. The archetype becomes activated and we become activated expressing whatever emotion is dominate. Othering in terms of raciality usually has the face of rage. This leads to aggression and the physical and/or mental harm of another. The African Holocaust is the circumstance which I have discussed in this book whereby shadow, racial complexes and othering compelled the destruction of millions of human lives.

We are living in times when we can influence the shadow archetype of racism. I believe that the election of President Barack Obama was the most significant proof of this in the 20th century. Just as we have collective influences of the archetype that has created a Jewish Holocaust, world wars, slavery, we also through human consciousness can respond in bringing to life that which reinforces our humanity. We are capable through conscious effort to reverse that which is of the shadow of racism and is destructive to our humanity and therefore our divinity. As we have learned more about our connections through socialization and social bonds, we know that fulfilling the needs of the ego alone is insufficient for preventing discrimination against others. We have learned that it is through "getting to know" others that we can develop empathy for them. This empathy can become love. "A simple fact of life, with profound neural consequences and mental health implications, is that we become attached to—we love—those who nurture and befriend us" (Panksepp and Biven, 2012, p. 313).

In speaking about our influence over the archetypes I am also speaking about our influence over our own individual behavior. I am addressing the need to see *something* which is beyond the limited ego's desire to have power and control over others. This type of control most often brings us only to unnatural deaths because of killing and large-scale wars. The agreement among nations to cease developing nuclear weapons is I believe a result of human consciousness touched by the divine in service of deepening a connection with the spirit of love, rather than hate. In moments of reflection, the collective is capable of influencing archetypal patterns that exist for destruction as well as good. Jung comments on the impartiality of the unconscious. We can see this at work in our society. Influencing the archetypes requires self-reflection, emotional effort and action. Just as the archetypes are patterns of potential action, we also become this through *activism*.

We cannot know with certainty which archetypal energy has even occurred in our collective memories that demands for us to engage with another in a destructive pattern. It does become obvious, however, that we can be with one another in a constructive archetypal pattern. The Abolitionist Movement was such an archetypal pattern as was the Civil Rights Movement of the 1960s. As we wrestle with what Sam Kimbles calls *social suffering*, we must think and feel into how we can influence invisible phantom forces which can either lead to a bettering of our lives or not. We do have the potential to remedy social suffering through a purposeful engagement with archetypal energy and patterns.

SUMMARY

When I began writing *Archetypal Grief: Slavery's Legacy of Intergenerational Child Loss*, I was deeply saddened for my ancestors and all of their descendants before me. As I read stories about their physical pain, torture and death through the generations it brought me into a different space of consciousness regarding the quality of life within my own cultural heritage. My recognition of what it took to bring me into this physical life, and all that might have been present on an archetypal level as my grandmother Rebecca brought me into the world with her midwifery skills, reflected the maternal lineage of my own mother and the mothers before her. My understanding of the means through which they must have struggled to survive on the plantations—from the beginning of Southern slavery auctions, until emancipation—greatly deepened as I read slave narratives. This was not only my own personal grief at their suffering but also the sacred honor at having been one of their descendants.

Archetypal Grief recognizes the accompanying sorrow that shows itself not only in the Africanist women who live today in a perpetual state of worry and concern for their male family members but also the historical pattern of abuse directed at African American men—sons, fathers, uncles, grandfathers. This caution and hyper-awareness for the safety of our male relatives has been developed over centuries. It cannot be denied that such an active state of attention is necessary. The reality also cannot be denied that large numbers of African American men have suffered shortened lives due to incarceration or violent death. This extended "watching over" and attention in the hope of keeping African American boys and men out of harm's way is also a legacy of slavery. It predicts how we will raise our children and the parenting styles dominant within our culture.

The *archetypal grief* of which I speak shows itself in my clinical practice with women of African ancestry and in my conversations with women friends and colleagues who are mothers and those who aren't. The latter are women who, fearful for the lives of their un-birthed children, have refused to birth these children into the world.

In the phenomenological field that holds us as we speak to one another, the sorrow of loss is strong and distinct. In the transference of this deep grief I understand and feel into the longevity of this grief. It is present in the room, in our bodies, showing itself almost visible as spirits coming once again to our place, a home of familiarity.

I propose that the *archetype of slavery* has its accompanying racial complexes that have kept our American racial conflicts alive in each new generation. The archetypal grief that Africanist women felt at being taken into slavery has been patterned and reformed over generations. The trauma of fear, anguish, rage, gets re-birthed with each new generation. This is the nature of archetypal cultural patterns. They become energized, enhanced, enlivened by environment, cultural factors and collective intentions whether they are positive or negative.

Paula Giddings describes some of the earliest days of parenting in *When and Where I Enter: The Impact of Black Women on Race and Sex in America*.

> The efforts of slave mothers to instill values in their children had an effect that was not always positive. The need to be exceedingly harsh or enterprising where their children were concerned often created emotional distance between mother and child. A slave by the name of Aunt Sally recalled how stern her mother was, "rarely talking with her children, but training them to be the best of her ability in all industry and honest." Every moment she could gain from labor, the narrator wrote, "was spent in spinning and knitting and sewing to keep them decently clothed." …. The tension was greater, noted slave Bethany Vency, when the child was a daughter, whose "almost certain doom is to minister to the unbridled lust of the slave owner." When Veney's daughter was born, she wished that both of them could "die right there and then." Such a wish is commonly expressed in the slave narratives of women, and a number of the rare but not insignificant instances of infanticide can be seen within this context.
>
> *(1988, p. 44)*

During the past three years, a greater number of deaths of African American men and women at the hands of law enforcement officers has been recorded than ever before in our recent history since the Jim Crow segregation era. In speaking of this in *Freedom Is a Constant Struggle: Ferguson, Palestine, and the Foundations of a Movement*, Angela Y. Davis says:

> Deep understandings of racist violence arm us against deceptive solutions. When we are told that we simply need better police and better prisons, we counter with what we really need. We need to reimagine security, which will involve the abolition of policing and imprisonment as we know them. We will say demilitarize the police, disarm the police, abolish the institution of the

police as we know it, and abolish imprisonment as the dominant mode of punishment. But we will have only just begun to tell the truth about violence in America.

(2016, p. 90)

This ability to see such tragic events, these deaths, in "real time" are mostly due to the latest designs in technology. In the not too distant "old days," African American men might have been brought to the precinct back room or sheriff's office and beaten or murdered. The only witnesses would have been the police, deputies and their associates.

African American men who have been victims of law enforcement attacks and murder have been filmed by phone cameras, video cameras and even police body cameras. The acknowledgement of this new technology offers little or no comfort to those of us who grieve with the family of the victims. However, it does offer us a view, a perspective, on how death can come so rapidly and seemingly without conscious humane recognition for the life of the victims. Most times, there has been no provocation and no reason for extreme force on the part of law enforcement officers. Victims have been found to have no weapons.

The recorded images of these assaults on African American men and boys have indeed become more frequently important in our conscious state. We rely on these images, and their presentation of truth that we find difficult to believe, even as we bear witness to such events. This contemporary perspective of African American men being harmed by law enforcement officers can mirror the elimination of them through incarceration. The underlying unconscious American collective pattern of "feeling" a need to contain, to control these male members of our society, continues centuries after the official end of slavery.

There appears to be no end to the attempted implementation of slavery in some form or another. Forces, ideas, commitment to harming African American men and women appears to continue as part of the American collective racial psyche. This type of harm revolves around the shadow of racism. Within the last century there have been more writings and conversations regarding society's racial unintentional and intentional harm, but the forces assertively pushing "enslavement" of some kind remain at work. When I say forces I'm considering the archetypal energy that I call *archetypal possession*—that overcomes us and makes us injure, love, or hate one another. This is part of the emotional energy that wishes to inflict pain or destruction on another because of skin color and *othering*.

What is this energy? Is it truly archetypal and can it be stopped or changed? What defines it in our American collective psyche? What would it mean to even consider eliminating thoughts and images of killing another? Murder and violence make an appearance in one of the first books—the Bible—in the story of Cain and Abel.

We appear to have a pattern for committing violent acts against each other. Is this an archetypal pattern and if so how do we influence it to allow ourselves to have peaceful relationships? Is this possible? There is a strong relationship between the archetypal grief of African American women and the painful pattern that we continue to see and feel in the violent deaths of African American sons, fathers and brothers. This is partly due to the refusal of our collective to consistently accept one another *not* as "Opposites" or "Others" as understood in a classical Jungian sense. The language of separation and segregation thrives as we struggle through what appears at time futile attempts to be with one another in peaceful relationships, letting go of "race" as the main determinant for how we might live together as members of the *human race*.

Jungian psychology, also known as analytical psychology, has as one of its core theories, the concept of the "Opposites." I think that when this concept is allowed to thrive unexamined, as it has been in our multicultural society, it supports racial dissension between us as varying ethnic groups. It has in our collective attached great ideals and emotional charge to the *racial Opposite*. The Swiss homogenous society in which Jung developed this theory of the "Opposites" creates more racial unrest in our diverse 21st century American society when left unexamined.

Of course, Jung is not responsible for our continued negative racial relationship that stagnates due to archetypes and complexes. Jung's apparent understanding of human psychology has in fact provided us with some of our most important and valued ideas and language for self-exploration of racism. It will be partly through a Jungian and post-Jungian lens discussed in this book that we will perhaps find some of the keys to our understanding of archetypal grief. However, there are other places for us to extend our search for the essential make-up of archetypal grief as well as grounding it in its historical past. We seek knowledge allowing archetypal grief to develop the fluidity it requires to receive our imprint of recognition and change which is centuries overdue. Some of these depthful places are familiar. Elisabeth Kubler-Ross speaks of the rite and rituals of death and mourning. The African Holocaust as experienced through slavery had centuries of this which we will have to revisit as many times as we can bear in order to see, re-vision and change our perspectives on relating in a different way than *othering*.

In the latest developments of neuroscience and neurobiology, 21st-century explorations of how we are connected to one another, examine brain structures and the relationship between us as human beings based on emotions and social environment. How do the archetypes influence our lives when epigenetics is a factor? Does a relationship exist between archetypes and epigenetics? What might this relationship be or become? Does chronological time change what we know about archetypes and their existence as Jung thought of them in the 19th century in light of our new knowledge regarding human neuroscience? These questions are part of the way we could inspect, re-live and reimagine the experiences of the intergenerational trauma of slavery, child breeding, and the grief of mothering slaves and their descendants.

In *Archetypal Grief: Slavery's Legacy of Intergenerational Child Loss*, we travel together into both familiar and unknown territories. How often have we considered slavery as an archetype?

We know grief and suffering because it is a defining aspect of being human. When have we last read a slave narrative and cried, trying to understand this level of suffering? In the 21st century, we continue to live through the suffering that slavery has brought to us but perhaps for many, it is a past best left there. The grief from this archetypal event has been explored in *Archetypal Grief* so that we—all of us—can deepen our understanding of what is demanded of us on life's journey. History matters. The historical fact of American slavery and cultural trauma lives in the psyches of African American women and men. It still calls out on an archetypal intergenerational level. How can we respond, attempting to meet this call, in that place where we can successfully influence the archetypes, and encourage healing on just as powerful a cultural and collective level?

If grief is possible so is resiliency. This is my hope for all that we must bear.

REFERENCES

American Buddhist Academy (1966). *The Teaching of Buddha (The Buddhist Bible)*. Tokyo: Kenkyusha Printing Co.
Anderson, C. (2017). *White Rage: The Unspoken Truth of Our Racial Divide*. London: Bloomsbury.
Bailey, A. C. (2017). *The Weeping Time: Memory and the Largest Slave Auction in American History*. New York: Cambridge University Press.
Baldwin, J. (1965). "Sonny's Blues," in *Going to Meet the Man*. New York: Dial Press.
Blassingame, J. W. (1972). *The Slave Community: Plantation Life in the Antebellum South*. New York and Oxford: Oxford University Press.
Bowlby, J. (1973). *Attachment and Loss: Separation Anxiety and Anger*. New York: Basic Books.
Bowlby, J. (1980). *Attachment and Loss: Sadness and Depression*. New York: Basic Books.
Brewster, Fanny. (2011). *The Dreams of African American Women: A Heuristic Study of Dream Imagery*. Ann Arbor, MI: Pro Quest UMI Dissertation Publishing.
Brewster, Fanny (2012). "Kensho: The Mirror of Self-Reflection," *Quadrant* 42(1):49–65.
Brewster, Fanny (2013). "Wheel of Fire: The African American Dreamer and Cultural Consciousness," in *Jung Journal: Culture and Psyche* 7(1): 70–85.
Brewster, Fanny (2017). *African Americans and Jungian Psychology: Leaving the Shadows*. London: Routledge.
Bynum, Edward Bruce. (2012). *The African Unconscious: Roots of Ancient Mysticism and Modern Psychology*. New York: Cosimo Books.
Davis, A. Y. (2016). *Freedom Is a Constant Struggle: Ferguson, Palestine, and the Foundations of a Movement*. Chicago, IL: Haymarket Books.
Davis, D. B. (2006). *Inhuman Bondage: The Rise and Fall of Slavery in the New World*. New York: Oxford University Press.
DeGruy, Joy. (2005). *Post Traumatic Slave Syndrome: America's Legacy of Enduring Injury and Healing*. Portland, OR: Joy DeGruy Publications.
DeHeusch, L. (1982). *The Drunken Kind or the Origin of the State*. Bloomington: Indiana University Press.

Equiano, Olaudah (1791). *The Interesting Narrative of the Life of Olaudah Equiano, Written by Himself*. Ed. Robert J. Allison. New York: W. Durell. Reprint, Boston, MA: Bedford Books, 1995.

Eyerman, R. (2001). *Cultural Trauma: Slavery and the Formation of African American Identity*. New York: Cambridge University Press.

Fordham, M. (1985). "Abandonment in Infancy," in *Chiron: A Review of Jungian Analysis*. Wilmette, IL: Chiron Publications.

Gates, H. L. (1988). *The Signifying Monkey: A Theory of African American Literary Criticism*. New York: Oxford University Press.

Giddings, Paula. (1988). *When and Where I Enter: The Impact of Black Women on Race and Sex in America*. New York: Bantam.

Gottlieb, A. (2004). *The Afterlife Is Where We Come From: The Culture of Infancy in West Africa*. Chicago, IL andLondon: University of Chicago Press.

Gudaite, G. and Stein, Murray. (2014). *Confronting Cultural Trauma: Jungian Approaches to Understanding and Healing*. New Orleans, LA: Spring Journal Books.

Guthrie, R. (2004). *Even the Rat Was White: A Historical View of Psychology*. Boston, MA: Pearson Education.

Guy-Sheftall, B. (1995). *Words of Fire: An Anthology of African-American Feminist Thought*. New York: The New Press.

Harris-Perry, V. M. (2011). *Sister Citizen: Shame, Stereotypes, and Black Women in America*. New Haven, CT andLondon: Yale University Press.

Hillman, J. (1983). *Archetypal Psychology: A Brief Account*. Dallas, TX: Spring Publications.

Herskovits, M. J. ([1958] 1990). *The Myth of the Negro Past*. Boston, MA: Beacon Press.

Hogenson, G. (2009). "Archetypes as Action Patterns," in *Journal of Analytical Psychology*, 54: 325–337.

Jablonka, E. and Lamb, M. J. (2014). *Evolution in Four Dimensions: Genetic, Epigenetic, Behavioral, and Symbolic Variation in the History of Life*. Cambridge, MA, and London: MIT Press.

Jacobi, J. ([1959] 1971). *Complex Archetype Symbol in the Psychology of C.G. Jung*. Princeton, NJ: Princeton University Press.

James, George G. M. (1992). *Stolen Legacy: Greek Philosophy Is Stolen Egyptian Philosophy*. Trenton, NJ: Africa World Press.

Jones, J. (2010). *Labor of Love, Labor of Sorrow: Black Women, Work, and the Family, from Slavery to the Present*. New York: Basic Books.

Joyner, C. (1984). *Down by the Riverside: A South Carolina Slave Community*. Urbana and Chicago: University of Illinois Press. Jung, C. G. ([1934] 1960). "A Review of the Complex Theory," in *The Structure and Dynamics of the Psyche*. The Collected Works. Vol. 8. R. F. C. Hull (trans.). Princeton, NJ: Princeton University Press.

Jung, C. G. ([1934] 1968). *The Archetypes and the Collective Unconscious*. The Collected Works, Vol. 9i. R. F. C. Hull (trans.). Princeton, NJ: Princeton University Press.

Jung, C. G. ([1959] 1973). *Four Archetypes: Mother/Rebirth/Spirit/Trickster*. Princeton, NJ: Princeton University Press.

Jung, C. G. (1973). *Memories, Dreams, Reflections*. New York: Random House.

Jung, C. G. (2009). *The Red Book: Liber novus*. New York: W. W. Norton.

Kendi, I. X. (2016). *Stamped from the Beginning: The Definitive History of Racist Ideas in America*. New York: Nation Books.

Kimbles, Samuel L. (2014). *Phantom Narratives: The Unseen Contributions of Culture to Psyche*. Lanham, MD: Rowman & Littlefield.

Knapp, R. J. (1986). *Beyond Endurance: When a Child Dies*. New York: Schocken Books.

Knox, J. (2012). *Archetype, Attachment, Analysis: Jungian Psychology and the Emergent Mind*. Hove: Routledge.

Kübler-Ross, E. (1970). *On Death and Dying*. New York: Macmillan.
Kübler-Ross, E. and Kessler, D. (2014). *On Grief and Grieving: Finding the Meaning of Grief Through the Five Stages of Loss*. New York: Scribner.
Leeming, D. (1996). *Goddess: Myths of the Female Divine*. New York: Oxford University Press.
Levy-Bruhl, L. (1960). *How Natives Think*. New York: Washington Square Press.
Lincoln, C. E. and Mamiya, H. (1990). *The Black Church in the African American Experience*. Durham, NC: Duke University Press.
Lowinsky, N. R. (1992). *The Motherline*. San Francisco, CA: Fisher King Press.
Maxwell, K. (1983). *Bemba Myth and Ritual: The Impact of Literacy on an Oral Culture*. New York: Peter Lang.
Mbiti, J. S. (1989). *African Religion and Philosophy*. 2nd ed. Portsmouth, NH: Heinemann Publishers.
Meaney, M. and Francis, D. (2002). *Maternal Care and the Development of Stress Responses in Foundations of Social Neuroscience*. Cambridge, MA: MIT Press.
Mellon, J. (ed.) (1988). *Bullwhip Days: The Slaves Remember*. New York: Grove Press.
Moore, D. S. (2015). *The Developing Genome: An Introduction to Behavioral Epigenetics*. New York: Oxford University Press.
Nanamoli, B.and Bodhi, B. (trans.) (2005). *The Middle Length Discourses of the Buddha*. Boston, MA: Wisdom Publications.
Neimark, P. (1993). *The Way of the Orisha: Empowering Your Life through the Ancient African Religion of Ifa*. New York: HarperCollins.
Nichols, E. (2015). "African American Funeral and Mourning Customs in South Carolina." *South Writ Large: Stories, Arts and Ideas from the Global South*, Fall. Available at www. Southwritlarge.com.
Panksepp, J. and Biven, L. (2012). *The Archeology of Mind: Neuroevolutionary Origins of Human Emotions*. New York and London: W. W. Norton & Company.
Piggott, J. (1969). *Japanese Mythology*. London: Hamlyn Publishing Group.
Puckett, Newbell (1926). *Folk Beliefs of the Southern Negro*. Chapel Hill, NC: Chapel Hill Press.
Rankin, C., LoffredaB. and Cap, K. (2015). *The Racial Imaginary: Writers on Race in the Life of the Mind*. New York: Fence Books.
Rizzolatti, G.and Sinigaglia, C. (2008). *Mirrors in the Brain: How our minds share Actions and Emotions*. New York: Oxford University Press.
Roberts, D. (2017). *Killing the Black Body: Race, Reproduction and the Meaning of Liberty*. New York: Penguin Random House.
Roediger, D. (2014). *The Wages of Whiteness*. Brooklyn, NY: Verso.
Ronnberg, A. (ed.) (2010). *The Book of Symbols: Reflections on Archetypal Images*. The Archive for Research in Archetypal Symbolism (ARAS). Cologne: Taschen.
Rosenblatt, P. C. and Wallace, B. R. (2005). *African American Grief*. New York and Hove: Routledge.
Savage, J. A. (1989). *Mourning Unlived Lives: A Psychological Study of Childbearing Loss*. Wilmette, IL: Chiron Publications.
Schwartz, M. J. (2009). *Birthing a Slave: Motherhood and Medicine in the Antebellum South*. Cambridge, MA: Harvard University Press.
Sertima, I. V. (Ed.) (1997). *Black Women in Antiquity*. New Brunswick, NJ and London: Transaction Publishers.
Sjoo, M. and Mor, B. (1987). *The Great Cosmic Mother: Discovering the Religion of the Earth*. San Francisco: HarperCollins.
Sterling, D. (ed.) (1984). *We Are Your Sisters: Black Women in the Nineteenth Century*. Markham, ON: Penguin Books.

Stewart, J. B. (1997). *Holy Warriors: The Abolitionists and American Slavery*. New York: Hill and Wang.
Sublette, N. and Sublette, C. (2016). *The American Slave Coast: A History of the Slave-Breeding Industry*. Chicago, IL: Lawrence Hill Books.
Temples, P. (1945). *Bantu Philosophy*. Paris: Présence Africaine Publishers.
Thelen, E. and Smith, L. B. (1996). *A Dynamic Systems Approach to the Development of Cognition and Action*. Cambridge, MA and London: MIT Press.
Tronick, E. (1986). *Maternal Depression and Infant Disturbance (New Directions for Child and Adolescent Development)*. San Francisco, CA: Jossey-Bass.
Vasconcellos, C. "Children in the Slave Trade," in *Children and Youth in History*, Item #141. Available at http://chnm.gmu.edu/cyh/items/show/141 (accessed June 3, 2018).
Von Franz, M. L. (1980). *Projection and Re-Collection in Jungian Psychology*. Peru, IL: Open Court Publishing.
Washington, H. (2008). *Medical Apartheid: The Dark History of Medical Experimentation on Black Americans from Colonial Times to the Present*. New York: Random House.
Webber, T. L. (1978). *Deep Like the Rivers: Education in the Slave Quarter Community, 1831–1865*. New York and London: W.W. Norton & Company.
White, D. G. (1998). *Ar'n't I a Woman? Female Slaves in the Plantation South*. New York: W. W. Norton & Company.
Williams, C. (1987). *The Destruction of Black Civilization: Great Issues of a Race from 4500 B.C. to 2000 A.D.* Chicago, IL: Third World Press.
Willis, R. (ed.) (1993). *Mythology: An Illustrated Guide*. London: Duncan Baird Publishers.
Wippler, M. G. (1989). *Santeria: The Religion*. New York: Harmony Books.

INDEX

Abandonment in Infancy (Fordham) 11
Abolitionist movement 35–7, 69, 108, 117, 119, 133
acceptance, as stage of grief 65–7
activism 133
Adams, John Quincy 37
African American Funeral and Mourning Customs in South Carolina (Nichols) 26–7
African American men: incarceration of xvi, 61, 79, 134, 136; violence against 134, 135–6; *see also* African Americans; slaves
African American women 5; angry xvi–xvii, 70, 74–9, 81; bearing sorrow 113–15; death of xx; empowerment of 117; as healers 111; health of 86–9; history of 110; as jezebel 45–6, 100, 116; as mammy 45–7, 100, 116; pregnant 16, 18, 87, 110, 113–15; punishment of 110; and racial complex 79–81; sexual assault of 42, 45, 69–70, 75–6, 77, 80, 104, 110, 113, 114, 118; stigmatization of 68–9; and welfare 116–17; *see also* African Americans; mothering slaves; grief; slaves
African Americans: anger of 60–1; attempted invisibility of 113; childbirth customs 14, 18–19; collective consciousness of xvii; collective past of 75; consciousness of 73; cultural complexes of xvi, 73–4; devaluation of 30; "emotionalism" of 71; false history of 73; need for expression 72; as "pre-logical" 71; silencing of 72; struggle for respect 84; *see also* African American men; African American women; slavery; slaves
African cultures xii, 18, 59, 97, 104–5
African customs 26, 81, 89, 103, 104, 112
African diaspora 4, 14, 22, 25, 26, 34, 38, 128; and acceptance of slavery 65–6; anger in 60; bargaining and death 61–2; children of 52; collective cultural suffering of 91–2; cultural differences 23; cultural trauma of 61; and the female body 115–17; funeral rituals of 56; on grieving and death 58; skin care issues 23; women of 116–17; *see also* African Americans; slaves
African history 98, 100
African Holocaust xx, 3, 28, 43, 51, 81, 95, 98, 128, 133; and the deaths of children 90; genocidal nature of 48; historical facts of 91; and the archetype of slavery 100; *see also* genocide; slavery
Africanist people *see* African American men; African American women; African Americans; African diaspora
African Religion and Philosophy (Mbiti) 14, 21, 56, 107
African spiritual traditions 12, 89
African Unconscious: Roots of Ancient Mysticism and Modern Psychology (Bynum) 9
afterlife belief 19, 23
Afterlife Is Where We Come From, The (Gottlieb) 18

alchemy 10
American Anti-Slavery Society 36
American Civil War *see* Civil War
American Revolution 35, 63
Amistad mutiny 37
analytical psychology 72, 137; *see also* Jungian psychology
ancestors: experience of 52, 73, 83, 105; generational listing of 51; honoring 31, 73; and the importance of funeral rituals 56; respect for 21, 115; as source of psychic energy 108–9; voice of 35–7
ancestral cult 19, 24, 25, 58
ancestral DNA 34, 117
Angelou, Maya xix
anger xvi–xvii, 3, 16–17; black 60–1; of black women xvi–xvii, 70, 74–9, 81; and grief 60–1, 68, 77; and mourning 93; repressed 81; as stage of grief 60–1
Angola 111
anthropologists 71
anxiety 16–17
Archeology of Mind, The: Neuroevolutionary Origins of Human Emotions (Panskepp and Biven) 130
archetypal DNA xxi, 5, 26, 60, 78, 81
archetypal possession 136
archetypal psychology 5; *see also* psychology
Archetype, Attachment, Analysis: Jungian Psychology and the Emergent Mind (Knox) 5–6
archetypes: Africanist 25; and the collective unconscious 1–3; cultural aspects of 2, 3–4, 31, 131; and the divine 5; of freedom 15; and imagery making 5; as image schema 6, 10; influence of 127, 132–3; Jung's theory of xvi, 31; models for defining 129; mother 4–5, 8–9; Mother of Sorrow xiii, 8–9, 90, 91; as a pattern 5; as psycho-spiritual entities 5; as representation of the divine 131; shape-taking ability of 5; of slavery 135, 137; as a type of energy 5, 10; of the way 92
Archetypes and the Collective Unconscious, The (Jung) 1
Ar'n't I a Woman: Female Slaves in the Plantation South (White) 44, 80
Attachment and Loss (Bowlby) 14
attachment disorders xxi
attachment theory xxi, 6, 14–17, 128, 130
At the Dark End of the Street: Black Women, Rape and Resistance (McGuire) 75–6

babies, in the Beng community 19–21
Bailey, Anne C. 78

Bakongo people 26
Baldwin, James xv, xix
bargaining, as stage of grief 61–3
Beloved (Morrison) xix
Bemba culture 102
Beng people 18, 95; life of babies 19–21
bestiality 44–5
Beyond Myth and Ritual. The Impact of Literacy on an Oral Culture (Maxwell) 102
Birney, James 36
Birthing a Slave: Motherhood and Medicine in the Antebellum South (Schwartz) 82, 87
birthing traditions 86–7
birth rituals: ear piercing 20; placenta burial 14; savanna grass necklace 20; and the umbilical cord 18–19, 20
Biven, Lucy 130
Black Church in the African American Experience, The (Lincoln and Mamiya) 12
Black Madonnas 100
Black Power movement 42, 45, 60, 119
black women: in Africa 111–12; as chiefs 111; *see also* African American women
body: black female xiii, xxi, 113–14, 117; connection to mind 115, 129, 131; connection to spirit 87; consciousness of 123; of a dead person 54–56, 58; as *defectus incubus* 94; emotional xxi, 105; freedom of 39, 117–18; healing 117; as narrative 115–17; reflection of 122; spirit- 125
Bonner, Lewis 37
Book of Symbols, The: Reflections on Archetypal Images (Ronnberg) 120–1
Bowlby, John 14, 15, 19, 92, 130
BrainMind functions 130
Brown, John 37
Brown, William Wells 85, 107
Buddhism 121–3, 132
Bynum, Edward Bruce 9–10

Cannady, Fanny 57–8, 59, 62, 70–1
Cannon, Norman 76
childbirth customs 14, 18–19
children: of the African diaspora 52; anxiety and hostility of 16; cognitive development of 11, 71; daughters 101–5; death of 82–3, 92–3, 94, 95; dreams of 83; health of 86–9; as intergenerational orphans 48–53; involved in death rituals 55–6; lost due to slavery 52, 82, 93, 94; murdered 94; physical and emotional state of 16; protection of 5, 15; sadness of 16; sons 105–9; susceptibility to death 21; traumatic loss of 11, 14–15; women's

fears related to xxi–xxii, 5, 74, 134–5; *see also* slave children
Christianity 4, 14, 132
circle, in mortuary traditions 27
circle dances 27
circumcision 107
cisungu ritual 102–3
civil liberties 61, 119
Civil Rights movement 42, 133
Civil War 37, 112
Coates, Rosa Lee 76
cognitive development, intergenerational 71
cognitive science 6, 7, 130
collective unconscious 1–3, 5, 128, 131
compassion, absence of 63
Complex Archetype Symbol (Jacobi) 5
complexes xv; in the unconscious 2; *see also* cultural complexes
confusion, and mourning 93
consciousness: African 22, 24, 59, 65–6, 73, 109, 115, 119; collective xvii, 23, 45, 64, 89; cultural 31, 34, 66, 83, 89, 91; ego 31, 123; human 1–2, 5, 10, 31, 38, 39, 52, 91, 95, 98, 121, 123, 128, 131, 133; individual xvi, 2; normal xv; public xii; racial 75; theory of 115
crying 93, 94
cultural collective 37, 77, 78, 83, 84, 105, 124, 126, 132
cultural complexes xvi, 79–81, 91; African American xvi, 73–4; Africanist 95
cultural heritage 26–7, 33
cultural past 83–4
culture: Africanist 3–4; archetypal energy of 100; Buddhism 4; Eurocentric 3–4, 33; skin as 24; yoga 4

daughters 101–5; *see also* children
David, Jonathan C. 27
Davis, Angela Y. 22, 135–6
Davis, David Brion 24, 38, 43, 69
death: American cultural approach to 54–5; avoidance of 23; of children 94; fear of 54–5; and the future 21–2; Kübler-Ross's stages of 57–67; myths about 95; as release from suffering 58–9, 62, 95; of slaves 70–1, 95
death rituals: funeral rites 25–6; involving children 55–6; involving the living-dead 56
Deep Like the Rivers: Education in the Slave Quarter Community, 1831–1865 (Webber) 85, 105
DeGruy, Joy 66
De Heusch, Luc 102

denial, as stage of grief 58–9
depression 5; and mourning 93; as stage of grief 63–5
depth psychology 31–4, 55
Destruction of Black Civilization, The: Great Issues of a Race from 4500 B. C. to 2000 A. D. (Williams) 97
Dickinson, Emily 113
Douglass, Frederick 84, 106, 109
Dowd, Maureen 47
dreams 1–3, 20, 32, 34, 52, 73, 83, 89, 93, 101, 123–4, 131
Dreams of African American Women, The: Heuristic Study in Dream Imagery 101
dream-soul 89
Dubois, W. E. 75
Dynamic Systems Approach to the Development of Cognition and Action, A (Thelen and Smith) 129

ear piercing 20
ego work 10
Egypt 97, 98; archetypal history of 111
Elkins, Stanley 38
emotional body xxi, 105; *see also* body
emotionalism 71
emotional learning 129
empathy 133
Enlightenment 35, 63
epigenetics 11, 129, 130, 137
Equiano, Olaudah 49
Esu (Legba) 12
Ethiopia 97
Even the Rat Was White: A Historical View of Psychology (Guthrie) 44

fear: of anger 60; anticipatory 5, 116; for children's safety 74, 106, 134–5; of the dark 32; of death 54; hidden xxi; of the masses 32; among plantation owners 37, 63, 117; of those in slavery 58, 90–1; trauma of 90, 135
fertility 4, 13, 14, 89, 104, 116
First Mother 96–7
Fordham, Michael 11
Four Archetypes: Mother/Rebirth/Spirit/Trickster (Jung) 2
freedom: and the Abolitionist movement 35–7; as archetype 37–40, 106, 108; of the body 117–18; imagination of 32; of the mind 118; psychological xiv, xviii, 45; of the spirit 118–19; struggle for 22–3, 60
Freedom is a Constant Struggle: Ferguson, Palestine, and the Foundations of a Movement (Davis) 22, 135–6

Freeman's Bureau 37, 119
Freud, Sigmund 10
funeral rites 25–6

Gaffney, Mary 58–9
Garrison, William Lloyd 36
Garvey, Marcus 119
Gates, Henry Louis, Jr. 12
genocide 22, 48, 66, 77, 81, 95; *see also* African Holocaust
German Holocaust 128, 133
Ghana 111
Giddings, Paula 69, 135
goddesses 4–5, 8–11, 99–102, 111; African 100; Hathor 121; Mami Wata 120–1; mothers as 126; Oshun 4, 13, 117
Gonzalez-Wippler, Migene 4
Gottlieb, Amy 18, 19–20
grave objects 26
grave rituals 26
Great Awakening 35–6
grief: and acceptance 65–7; as anger 60–1, 68, 77; anticipatory 58; archetypal 4, 7, 10, 11, 26, 28–9, 52, 89–95, 100, 105, 130, 134–5, 137; authentic 83; and bargaining 61–3; of black women 47; and death 77; and denial 58–9; and depression 63–5; emotional inheritance of 27; and guilt 90, 93; hidden 68–73; intergenerational patterning of xix, 7, 52; of mothers 95; psychological xiii; and rage 94; and slavery 3; and the stages of death 57–67; and suffering 138; *see also* mourning; sadness; sorrow
guilt, and grief 90, 93
Gullah people 112
Guthrie, Robert V. 44

Haiti 71
Han, Thich Nhat 32
Harris-Perry, Melissa V. 42–3, 47, 116
healing xiii, xv, 63, 64–5, 84, 88, 92, 112, 117, 121, 138; collective xvii, 52; group 64, mother of 120; racial 53
Heming, Sarah 45, 69
Henderson, Joseph xv
Herskovits, Melville J. 55, 104; "Africanisms in Secular Life" 14; *The Myth of the Negro Past* 23–4, 25, 89, 103
Hillman, James xvii–xviii
Hogenson, George 128
How Natives Think (Levy-Bruhl) 71

Ifa 12–13
image schema 10

imagination 6, 10, 31
immediatists 36
immortality, personal 21–2
Indian culture 98
Individuation 33
Industrial Revolution 42
infertility 87, 89; *see also* fertility
Inhuman Bondage: The Rise and Fall of Slavery in the New World (Davis) 24, 69
initiation rituals: for boys 107–8; for girls 101, 102–3

Jacobi, Jolande 5
Jefferson, Thomas 35, 45, 69
Jewish Holocaust 128, 133
Jews, persecution of 127
jezebel stereotype 45–6, 100, 116
Jim Crow segregation 60, 119, 128
Johanson, Donald 115
Jones, Jacqueline 69–70
Jones, Thomas 84–5
Jung, Carl: on Africanist people 128; on archetypes xv–xvi, 4, 5, 31, 127; "Aspects of the Feminine" 96; on the collective unconscious 1–3, 9, 31, 128, 131; on DNA 78; dream of Self 2–3, 124; Knox's discussion of 6; on mothers 10–11, 96; on mythology 124; on opposites 38; on participation mystique 115; on "splinter psyches" xv
Jungian psychology 4, 33, 72, 74–5, 83, 121, 128, 137

Kessler, David 57, 60, 78
Killing the Black Body: Race, Reproduction and the Meaning of Liberty (Roberts) 115
Kimbles, Samuel xii, xiv, xv, xxi, 3, 73, 91, 133
King, Martin Luther, Jr. xviii, 118, 119
kinship groups 109
Knox, Jean 5–6, 10, 31, 128, 129–30
Kübler-Ross, Elisabeth 77, 137; on anger 60, 78; and cultural awareness of death 54–6; on the stages of death 57–67
Ku Klux Klan 119

Labor of Love, Labor of Sorrow: Black Women, Work and the Family from Slavery to the Present (Jones) 70, 110
land, desire for closeness to 22
Lane, Lunsford 105–6
Legba (Esu) 12
Levi-Strauss, Claude 102
Lewis, J. Vance 84
Liberty Party 37

life force energy 24, 26
Lincoln, Abraham 37
Little, Joan 76
Loguen, Jermain 85
longing 92–3
love 133
Lowinsky, Naomi Ruth 99
Lucy (oldest hominid) 115
lynching 118, 119

Mack, Chaney 50
Malcolm X 119
Mami Wata 120–1
mammy stereotype 45–7, 100, 116
Mary mother of Jesus 9, 90; connection to Yemoja 13
masses, fear of 32–3
Maxwell, Kevin 102
Mbiti, John S. 14, 21, 56, 107
McGuire, Danielle L. 76
medical doctors 87–8
Memories, Dreams, Reflections (Jung) 2, 92, 124
memory: archetypal 81; collective xx, 75, 83, 112, 117; implicit 6; importance of xxi; phantom xxiii; racial 9–10
Middle Length Discourses of the Buddha, The 121–2
Middle Passage 26, 42, 68, 73, 75, 81, 82, 90, 94, 100, 112
midwives 86–7
mirroring, psychic 123–4
mirror neurons 6, 10, 59, 71, 128, 129, 131–2
mirrors: in Japanese mythology 125–6; of self-reflection 121–2; as symbol 120–1
Mirrors in the Brain: How Our Minds Share Actions and Emotion (Rizzolatti and Sinigaglia) 6
missionaries 71
Moore, Roy 64
Morrison, Toni xix
mother archetype 4–5, 8–9
mothering slaves xxii, 41–2, 70, 94; and cultural rituals 101; descendants of 132, 137; emotional lives of 94–5, 104–5; as goddess-mother 126; *see also* mothers; slaves
"Mothering Slaves: Maternity, Childlessness and the Care of Children During and After Slavery" (2016 Conference) 41
Motherline, The (Lowinsky) 99
mother of Moses 9
Mother of Sorrow archetype xiii, 8–9, 90, 91
Mother of the Ocean *see* Yemoja/Yemaya

mothers: archetypal 100; and daughters 101–5; enslaved 15–17; fearing for children's safety xxi–xxii, 5, 74, 134–5; First Mother 96–7; group cohesiveness of 99; influence on child development 11; loss of children by 92–3; as mirror 126; personal 10–11; and sons 105–9; *see also* African American women; mothering slaves; women
Mother Water (Mami Wata) 120–1
mourning 3, 92–3; *see also* grief; sadness; sorrow
Mourning Unlived Lives: A Psychological Study of Childbearing Loss (Savage) 92
Myth of the Negro Past, The (Herskovits) 23–4, 25, 89, 103
mythologies 1, 3, 4, 5, 10; African 89–90; African Holocaust 11–13; and African initiation rites 101–2; creation 95, 102, 111–12, 121; of death 89–90, 95; goddess 99–100; Isis weeping 8–9, 90; Japanese 124–5; of the mirror 121–2; and the mother archetype 8–9; and ritual 102; Yoruba 12–13
Mythology: An Illustrated Guide 89–90

natural law 35
Neimark, Philip John 13
Neumann, Erich 92
neurobiology 11, 137
neurology, and the archetype 129
neuroscience xxi, 6–7, 10, 130, 137
"new slavery" 69
Nichols, Elaine 26
Nigeria, archetypal history of 111
Nihongi texts 124

Obama, Barack 47–8, 133
Obama, Michelle 47–8
Oberlin College 36
On Death and Dying (Kübler-Ross) 54–5, 57
On Grief and Grieving: Finding the Meaning of Grief Through the Five Stages of Loss (Kübler-Ross and Kessler) 57
Opposite(s) 61, 137; and the Opposite Other 79; racial 137
oral traditions 102, 103
Orisha 4, 12, 13
orphans, intergenerational 48–53; *see also* children
Oshun 4, 13, 117
Other(s) 137; anger and guilt of 77; demeaning of 81; in depth psychology 32; gendered xvi; grieving 60; Opposite 79; Self as 122–4; voice of 34; white 119
Owens, Betty Jean 76

pain: of the African American experience 136–7; and anger 60–1; cultural 53; emotional 66; and the human experience 7; of initiation rituals 107; and mourning 93; psychological 41; of slavery 28, 39, 41, 42, 62, 78, 96, 104, 134; understanding 68
Panskepp, Jaak 130
participation mystique 33, 115
Patterson, Orlando 38–9
Perkins, Gertrude 76
phantom memory xxiii
phantom narratives xv, xvii
Phantom Narratives: The Unseen Contributions of Culture to Psyche (Kimbles) xii, xiv, xxi, 3, 73, 91
placenta burial 14
polygamy 80
Post Traumatic Slave Syndrome: America's Legacy of Enduring Injury and Healing (DeGruy) 66
Post Traumatic Stress Syndrome 16
potentiality 4, 25, 31, 47, 52, 108, 126
process and change 129
psyche: African American 35, 64, 101, 119, 138; Africanist 52, 59, 95, 104, 115; American 42, 61, 64, 75; American collective 45, 98, 136; American collective racial 47, 136; American political 35; archetypal 74; of birthing mothers 11; energy of 129; human 130; Jung's concept of 2, 3, 4, 7; objective 123; personal 2; racialized American 116, 117; transformation of 32; unconscious xv, xviii, 30
psychic energy, through ancestral lineage 108
psychic mirroring 123–4
psychic wellness 105
psychological abandonment 51–2
psychology: analytical 72, 137; archetypal 5; depth 31–4, 55; Jungian 4, 33, 72, 74–5, 83, 121, 128, 137; of liberation 32
puberty rites 107
Puckett, Newbell 25, 55, 89

Quakers 35, 36, 117

racial complexes, 32, 116, 133, 135; and African American women 79–81
racial discrimination 34, 42
racism xviii; American 60–1, 64, 66, 69, 75; archetype of 133, 136; and the collective unconscious 128; and cultural trauma 53, 60; effects of 91, 96, 98, 113; and Jim Crow 60, 119, 128; Jungian discussion of 75, 137; opposition to 72; and physical difference 23, 24; and slavery 29, 61, 80, 113; and stereotypes 19, 75; and white supremacy 22, 76
rage: and aggression 133; and grief 94
Rahula (Buddha's son) 121–2
Red Book (Jung) 33
reincarnation xiv, 19–20
religion 10; African Methodist Episcopal 13; African spiritual traditions 21; Baptist 13; Buddhism 121–3, 132; Catholicism 13; charismatic 12; Christianity 4, 14, 132; Islam 12, 14; neo-Pentecostal 12; Pentecostal 12–13; Protestant 11–12; Santeria 4, 11, 13; Shinto 124; Taoism 132; and the unchurched 12; Voudou 4, 11
remembering 104–5; *see also* memory
reparations 29, 67
resiliency xxiii, 138
ring shouts 27
rites of passage: birth rituals 18–19, 23; death rituals 18, 23; interweaving of cultural patterns of 27
rituals: *cisungu* ritual 102–3; and myth 102; post-birth 14
Rizzolatti, Giacomo 6, 131
Roberts, Dorothy 115
Roediger, David R. xiv
Ronnberg, Ami 120

sadness 3, 5, 14, 16, 47, 64, 68, 77, 78, 93; *see also* grief; mourning; sorrow
"Sambo" ideology 38–9, 72
Santeria 4, 11, 13
Santeria: The Religion (Gonzalez-Wippler) 4
Savage, Judith A. 92, 94
savanna grass necklace 20
Schwartz, Marie Jenkins 82, 87
segregation 60, 118–19, 137
Self: alignment with 129; archetypal 2–3; Jung's dream of 2–3, 124; as Other 122–4
separation 2, 16, 17, 52, 102, 126, 137
Sessions, Jeff 64
shaming 42–3, 113
Sharpe, Granville 35
Signifying Monkey, The (Gates) 12
Sinigaglia, Corrado 6, 131
Sister Citizen: Shame, Stereotypes, and Black Women in America (Harris-Perry) 42–3, 116
slave auctions 34, 46, 49, 51, 62, 66, 78–9, 95, 134
slave children 15–16, 48–9, 84–6; born into slavery 51; psychological abandonment of

51–2; removed from slave parents 5, 93; stolen from Africa 50, 82; voices of 50–1; as witness to violence 16, 85; *see also* children; slave narratives
slave narratives 118, 134; Fanny Cannady 57–8, 59, 62; Ellen Cragin 72; Robert Farmer xxii; Mary Gaffney 58–9; Tom Hawkins 72; Charley Hurt 63; Lunsford Lane 105; J. Vance Lewis 84–5; Chaney Mack 50; Jack Maddox 50–1; Hester Norton 51; Katie Sutton 50; Harriet Tubman 15; Jennie Webb 50
slavery: abolition of in the British Empire 35; abolition of in France 35; abolition of in Haiti 71; abolition of in northern states 35; abolition of in the US 82, 118–19; and African spirituality 22; as archetypal event 60, 99, 100, 106, 135, 137; collective denial of 29–30; cultural trauma of 4–5, 77; and depression 63–4; and the destruction of families 30–1, 49, 51–2; and grief 78; harm done by xx–xxi, xxii, 4, 83, 116, 130; influence of 3, 11, 26; intergenerational 48; justifications for 64, 71; maternal lineage of 43–4, 84; nature of 28–31; "new" 69; in the New World 43–8; and the stages of grief 57–67; *see also* African Holocaust; mothering slaves; slave auctions
Slavery Abolition Act (Britain) 35
slaves: humane treatment of 69; restriction on speech of 70; training of 85–6; transportation of female 68–9; violence against 85; women as 69; *see also* African Americans; slave children
Smith, Linda B. 129, 131
social suffering 133
"Sonny's Blues" (Baldwin) xv, xix
sons 105–9; relationship with mothers 106
sorrow xx, 29, 49, 52, 56, 65, 78, 83, 91, 104, 134, 135; bearing 113–15; *see also* grief; sadness
spirituality, African-oriented 10, 11, 132
spiritual-mystical tradition 10
spiritual songs 118–19
spirit villages 18
splinter psyches xv
stereotypes: jezebel 45–6, 100, 116; mammy 45–7, 100, 116; Sambo 38–9, 72; *see also* African American women, angry
Sterling, Dorothy 15
Stewart, James Brewer 36
"Still I Rise" (Angelou) xix
St. Louis World Fair (1904) 44

Stroyer, Jacob 107
suffering: and grief 138; psychological 101; of slaves xiii; social 133; understanding xix

Taoism 132
Tappan, Lewis 36
Taylor, Recy 76
telos 1
Teng, Betty P. xiii
Thelen, Esther 129, 131
Thompson, Robert Ferris 26
time, concept of 21
transference 131–2
trauma: of abusive captivity 90–1; cultural 4, 42, 49, 59, 60, 61, 66, 77, 138; effect on brain function 130; and grief 90; intergenerational 17, 27, 49, 117, 128, 130, 135, 137; of slavery 28
tribal dances 80
Trump, Donald xii, xviii, 48, 60
Truth, Sojourner 12
Tubman, Harriet 12, 15
Turner, Nat 109

umbilical cord 18–19, 20; as charm 14

Vesey, Denmark 37
violence: against African-American men 134, 135–6; archetypal pattern of 136–7; ongoing 90–1; racist 135–6; sexualized 76; against slaves 85, 118; toward slaves xxii, 44, 51, 59, 62, 85, 130; witness by children 16, 85
Virgin Mary *see* Mary mother of Jesus
von Franz, Marie-Louise 123–4
Voting Rights Act (1965) 76
Voudou 4, 11

Wages of Whiteness, The (Roediger) xiv
Way of the Orisha, The (Neimark) 13
We Are Your Sisters: Black Women in the Nineteenth Century (Sterling) 15
Webber, Thomas L. 85, 106
Weeping Time, The: Memory and the Largest Slave Auction in American History (Bailey) 78
When and Where I Enter: The Impact of Black Women on Race and Sex in America (Giddings) 69, 135
White, Deborah Gray 44, 46, 80
White, Mingo 70
white nationalism 60, 118
white rage xviii, 60, 79, 117
white supremacy 22, 29, 64, 76
white women: elevation of 43, 45, 80; fears of 47; medical care for 88

Wilberforce, William 35
Williams, Chancellor 97
women: "barren" 87; as healers 86–8; and the mother archetype 4–5; pregnant 18–19, 22, 86–7, 115–16; role in ending slavery 119; and the work of remembering 104; *see also* African American women; mothering slaves; mothers; white women
Woolman, John 24

World's Congress of Races 44
Wright, Elizur 36

yearning 92–3
Yemoja 9
Yemoja/Yemaya 9, 13
Yoruba religious tradition 4, 12–13, 89, 99, 100, Yemoja/Yemaya 9, 13

Zamani 21